MAKE A DECISION: SURGERY

This book is dedicated entirely to my wife Elaine and my son Alex, without whom simply none of what I do would be either possible, or worthwhile.

MAKE A DECISION: SURGERY

MARK CORRIGAN
MB, BAO, BCh, BMedSci, MRCSI, MD
Royal College of Surgeons, Dublin, Ireland

PROFESSOR ARNOLD DK HILL
MCh, FRCSI
*Professor of Surgery, Royal College of Surgeons,
and Beaumont Hospital, Dublin, Ireland*

PROFESSOR HP REDMOND
MCh, FRCSI
*Professor of Surgery, University College Cork,
and Cork University Hospital, Cork, Ireland*

WILEY-BLACKWELL

A John Wiley & Sons, Ltd., Publication

This edition first published 2010, © 2010 by Mark Corrigan, Arnold DK Hill and
HP Redmond

Blackwell Publishing was acquired by John Wiley & Sons in February 2007.
Blackwell's publishing programme has been merged with Wiley's global Scientific,
Technical and Medical business to form Wiley-Blackwell.

Registered office: John Wiley & Sons Ltd, The Atrium, Southern Gate, Chichester,
West Sussex, PO19 8SQ, UK

Editorial offices: 9600 Garsington Road, Oxford, OX4 2DQ, UK
The Atrium, Southern Gate, Chichester, West Sussex, PO19 8SQ, UK
111 River Street, Hoboken, NJ 07030-5774, USA

For details of our global editorial offices, for customer services and for information
about how to apply for permission to reuse the copyright material in this book
please see our website at www.wiley.com/wiley-blackwell.

ISBN: 9781405196840

A catalogue record for this book is available from the British Library and the
Library of Congress.

Set in 9/12pt FF The Sans by Graphicraft Limited, Hong Kong
Printed and bound in Malaysia by Vivar Printing Sdn Bhd

1   2010

Contents

SECTION 1

What you're going to learn

What you might also learn

Case presentations

Perspectives

Investigations

SECTION 2

What you're going to learn

What you might also learn

Case presentations

Perspectives

Investigations

SECTION 3

What you're going to learn

What you might also learn

Case presentations

Perspectives

Investigations

Make a Decision Online

Acknowledgements

I would also like to express my debt and my gratitude to the many colleagues, friends and patients who have helped me directly and indirectly, in discussions, advice, support and in allowing me to participate in their care. In particular I would like to acknowledge the contribution of Mr. Daragh Moneley, consultant vascular surgeon, for his advice and particularly his critical appraisals.

Finally I would like acknowledge the co-authors of this book, Professors Paul Redmond and Arnold Hill for their continual encouragement, enthusiasm and mentorship.

Mark Corrigan

Introduction

Welcome to *Make a Decision: Surgery*. This book is designed to be a role-playing teaching aid for senior medical students and junior doctors, and represents a typical night on call or work day, in surgery. The reader takes on the role of Dr A Simpson, a junior doctor who is just starting a specialist career. Your job is to safely complete your night on call, prioritising, diagnosing and treating the patients you are referred. As sometimes happens in reality, help is not always to hand, and often you will have to make decisions armed with only the information you are given. Working in a hospital is far removed from the theory of textbooks, and this book has been designed to reflect this. Throughout the book, you will encounter characters typical of those seen in a large institution, some helpful and some not so helpful. Although core knowledge of the fundamentals is essential, hospitals are about people, primarily patients, staff and relatives. An inability to deal with people will make your clinical job impossible. Where practical, we have attempted to incorporate this into the book.

The book is divided into three sections of varying length, reflecting three breaks, or rest periods, within your shift. Before each section you will find the learning objectives expected from completing the section. Similarly, at the end of each section, you will be debriefed within the Perspectives section. This section is designed to dissect the scenarios you have completed and to incorporate evidence-based decisions into your approach. As you progress, your decisions will lead you to be awarded or deducted points – keep a score of these. At the end of the sections, and the book, you will find feedback according to the points scored. If a decision is especially dangerous, you may be 'dismissed' immediately. If you have been dismissed, you may restart the game at the beginning of the book or at the start of the next section.

At the end of each section you will find a short glossary of terms used. This will help explain some of the more unusual terms or disease categorisations used. Clinical experience is critical and as this book is made up of those cases which have taught us something important in our careers, we would encourage you to submit outlines of the cases that have impacted on you, along with the characters that you have encountered (good and bad) along the way. These can be submitted through the book's website at www.pilgrimshospital.com.

We hope that you enjoy *Make a Decision: Surgery*, and that it gives you an opportunity to encounter some of the problems you are guaranteed to face as a junior doctor on call. While not designed in any way to be a reference text, it is hoped that it may act as a stimulus for further reading in the various topics. Please do not try and learn the facts and figures we present to you; it is this rote learning approach to medicine that we are trying to discourage. Instead, use these facts and statistics as a stimulus to question your practice and strive for making your decisions evidence based. Some of the websites and resources we have found helpful over the years are recommended at the back of the book. Good luck!

Mark Corrigan
Arnold Hill
Paul Redmond

How to use this book

1. Each paragraph is numbered.

2. Start at paragraph 001.

3. At the end of each paragraph you will be instructed to turn to a new paragraph or given a series of choices. For example 'turn to 034' means you should turn to paragraph number 034.

4. Depending on your choices, you are awarded or deducted points. You should keep a record of your total.

5. The book is divided into three sections.

6. When you have finished the section you will be given feedback based on your score.

7. Also, after each section there is a perspectives section which will dissect the cases you have completed, giving you the evidence for your decisions.

8. At various stages of the book you will be told to check the blood or urine reports on your patients. These will be labelled with your patient's name and details, and are found at the end of this section in the Investigations.

9. After you have finished with Perspectives, move on to the next section of the book.

Introduction to the staff and nomenclature of Pilgrims Hospital

Staff

W. Halsted: The head surgeon
Ed Cahoon: Your senior
Mia Chang: Your intern
Nicola Pablo: Anaesthetist
Ruth Benedict: Radiologist
Margaret Hellman: Head nurse in the emergency department
Eileen, Joy, Ubeki, Caroline, Izzy: Nurses in the emergency department
Charles Winston: Your main competition in medical school and now in surgical training
Samuel Norman: The bed co-ordinator

Nomenclature

Pilgrims Hospital is a truly international institution and is not meant to reflect any particular country. However, the nature of medicine and surgery is that different countries and hospitals will have different terms for procedures, grades of staff, work practices, etc. To help with this, we have included a list of exchangeable nomenclature. If we have missed some you'll have to forgive us and let us know what they are.

The head surgeon: consultant, attending
Your senior (Ed Cahoon): registrar, resident
Intern: Foundation house officer, Foundation doctor, junior house officer
Emergency department: emergency room, accident and emergency, casualty
Head nurse: clinical nurse manager, sister, charge nurse
Medical school: university, college
Prescribe: chart
TDS: TID, three times daily
Rectal examination: digital rectal examination, DRE, PR examination
Round: ward round

SECTION 1

What you're going to learn

After this section you should be able to prioritise surgical patients in the setting of a busy accident and emergency department. Patients should be triaged according to threat to life, limb or organ, with those patients at highest risk treated first.

What you might also learn

Following completion of this section, you will be capable of performing the following in an evidence-based fashion.

• Using analgesia in the acute abdomen.
• Investigating and imaging the acute abdomen.
• Consider the conservative and operative management of the acute abdomen, including laparoscopic and open approaches.
• Adapt a sequential approach to trauma.
• Understanding and managing hypovolaemic shock and fluid resuscitation.
• Controlling simple postoperative bleeding.
• Managing superficial tissue infections.

Now, before you start, make sure you have read the background and the instructions.

16.40 SHIFT STARTS

It has been almost 3 months since the job offer arrived. The interview was tough – those old guys know how to hit you with some awkward questions – but you impressed them enough to get your first choice of hospital and your second choice of job. Pilgrims was one of the best surgical hospitals in the country, but recent cutbacks in government spending have hit even the biggest of institutions. You've just finished your first year after medical school and now your first rotation on the training scheme is with a busy general surgical firm and you are eager to impress. Your initial excitement was somewhat dampened upon hearing that Winston had received an identical offer. You competed neck and neck with Charles Winston through medical school but he narrowly beat you to first place in your final exams. You had hoped to put his smug face behind you, but now you will both be on the same training scheme, competing neck and neck once again. Only 8 hours into the job, you are faced with your first night on call. Your senior doctor, Ed Cahoon, will be on call with you along with the head surgeon

W. Halsted. Cahoon is in theatre with a difficult case that started several hours ago and you will have to face the start of your shift alone. Cahoon has a mean reputation, but nothing is going to dampen your enthusiasm for your first night on the job.

001 It's 5pm and your bleep goes off. Quickly finishing your dinner, you walk down the narrow corridor, passing the intensive care unit and the theatres and into the emergency department. Outside the main entrance, a stream of people queue to be seen and your heart races. The door to triage opens and you catch the eye of the triage nurse, surrounded by charts. Her face widens, the smile having no warmth. *'You're going to be busy tonight,'* she grins. Suddenly that skip in your step disappears and the automatic doors slide open to reveal the chaos behind them. You take a deep breath and roll up your sleeves before reaching for the two charts in the surgical slot.

> *I. A 14-year-old girl with vomiting and low abdominal pain* ⋯⟩ **012**

> *II. A 35-year-old man with cellulitis* ⋯⟩ **092**

002 You rightly choose the most potential serious case, **add 1 point**. Sharyn Romanowska, a 62-year-old lady with chronic inflammatory bowel disease, cardiac disease and COPD, presents with sudden onset of epigastric pain. In her past surgical history she has had a right hemicolectomy, open cholecystectomy and a small bowel resection for Crohn's disease more than 10 years ago. Her pulse is 130 and her BP 92/72. Sharyn's bloods are found in the Investigations at the end of this section. Currently she is sobbing with pain, lying absolutely still on the bed. Her elderly husband stands nervously in the corner of the resus room, insisting to you that it was the chicken she ate last night. *'I told her not to eat it, I told her'*. Do you:

> *I. Examine her* ⋯⟩ **038**

> *II. Get more of a history* ⋯⟩ **033**

> *III. Administer analgesia* ⋯⟩ **032**

> *IV. Order four units of blood urgently* ⋯⟩ **105**

> *V. Insert a second IV line* ⋯⟩ **053**

> *VI. Give more IV fluids* ⋯⟩ **011**

> *VII. Go to theatre for an exploratory laparotomy* ⋯⟩ **069**

> *VIII. Group and save her blood type for future possible blood cross-matching* ⋯⟩ **165**

003 You administer the prochlorperazine and within a short while she settles back. She tells you she has only a dull ache around her belly button. She has no urinary or bowel symptoms and this has never happened before.

   I. If you want to take a further history ⋯⟩ 065

   II. If you want to examine her ⋯⟩ 008

   III. If you want to look at her investigation results ⋯⟩ 118

   IV. If you want to order radiological tests ⋯⟩ 136

004 You administer the cyclizine and within a short while she settles back. She tells you she has only a dull ache around her belly button. She has no urinary or bowel symptoms and this has never happened before.

   I. If you want to take a further history ⋯⟩ 065

   II. If you want to examine her ⋯⟩ 008

   III. If you want to look at her investigation results ⋯⟩ 118

   IV. If you want to order radiological tests ⋯⟩ 136

005 It's a good idea to examine the patient where possible, before starting treatment. However, in this case your diagnosis is right. The man's urine output is reduced, his CVP is down, his urinary specific gravity is increased, his HCT is increased and his urea is increased with a normal creatinine. The picture is that of dehydration. You give him a fluid challenge of 500 ml over 30 minutes and his pulse slows to 88, BP rises to 134/76, urine climbs to 30 ml and CVP rises to 6. **Give yourself 1 point**. Do you:

   I. Recheck in 1 hour ⋯⟩ 058

   II. Check again in the morning ⋯⟩ 120

006 You get to the ward and see a relieved Mia holding the lady's leg at the end of the bed. **Add 1 point**. Her pulse is now 78 and her BP is 126/76. Mia tells you she had stripping of her long saphenous vein earlier today with stab avulsion of her varicosities. She takes her hand away and you see slow ooze from one of the stab avulsion sites on her calf. The staff nurse tells you that they have not needed to change the dressing until now. The dressings appear to have soaked up about 20 ml of blood. Do you:

   I. Take over from Mia and ask the nurses to call Cahoon ⋯⟩ 084

   II. Take over from the intern, raise the leg in the air and apply a compression dressing ⋯⟩ 086

   III. Get the intern to continue, raise the leg in the air and place a stitch at the avulsion site ⋯⟩ 139

   IV. Apply a tourniquet proximal to the bleeding point ⋯⟩ 148

007 The plain film of the abdomen is normal. **Deduct 1 point**.

I. If you want a chest x-ray ⋯⟩ 036

II. If you want an ultrasound abdomen ⋯⟩ 031

III. If you want a CT abdomen ⋯⟩ 112

008 You lay the girl down flat for examination.

I. If you want to tell her mother to stay and carry on examining her ⋯⟩ 051

II. If you want to tell her mother to leave and then examine her alone ⋯⟩ 154

III. If you want to ask her mother to leave and then bring in a nurse chaperone before examining her ⋯⟩ 115

009 You try to perform a laparoscopy but there are dense adhesions secondary to her two previous laparotomies and previously active Crohn's disease. You change to an open laparotomy and discover the bile-stained fluid of a perforated duodenum. You close this with an omental patch and the lady is returned to the ICU. Two days later she is transferred from the ICU to the ward and she eventually makes a full recovery. Well done, **add 1 point**.

Return to the surgical slot ⋯⟩ 067

010 The lady is diffusely tender with generalised guarding and rebound. Bowel sounds are absent and she is clammy to the touch. Her tongue is dry, fissured and cracked. Margaret is standing beside you and can't believe you're not going to theatre straight away. Do you next:

I. Get more of a history ⋯⟩ 099

II. Administer morphine ⋯⟩ 075

III. Get radiology ⋯⟩ 060

IV. Go to theatre for an exploratory laparotomy ⋯⟩ 069

011 Recognising that the lady is profoundly dehydrated, you administer IV fluids and insert a urinary catheter to monitor her output hourly. Within 30 minutes her pulse has slowed to 96 and her blood pressure has improved to 100/64. **Add 1 point**. Do you next:

I. Examine her ⋯⟩ 010

II. Get more of a history ⋯⟩ 099

III. Administer morphine ⋯⟩ 075

IV. Get radiology ⋯⟩ 060

V. Go to theatre for an exploratory laparotomy ⋯⟩ 089

012 You obviously prioritise your patients and she is the more likely to need surgery; **add 1 point**. You flick quickly through the girl's chart. Karen Twentyman is a 14-year-old girl with no medical history of note. Three days ago she developed mild suprapubic pain with associated nausea and vomiting. The triage nurse has sent off a urine sample for culture. You pull back the curtain and a stocky girl in a school uniform is vomiting into a kidney dish. Her mother rubs her back and looks up as you enter. Eileen, the nurse looking after her, asks you to prescribe an antiemetic in order to make the girl more comfortable.

> I. If you want to give her prochlorperazine ⋯⟩ **003**

> II. If you want to give her cyclizine ⋯⟩ **004**

> III. If you want to give her ondansetron ⋯⟩ **079**

> IV. If you want to hold off the antiemetics and try to elicit a history first ⋯⟩ **029**

013 She tells you that the patient has deteriorated and needs to be seen. Do you:

> I. Tell her you'll see her after you're finished with this patient ⋯⟩ **028**

> II. Go and see for yourself ⋯⟩ **077**

014 The lady is diffusely tender with generalised guarding and rebound. Bowel sounds are absent and she is clammy to touch. Her tongue is dry, fissured and cracked. Do you:

> I. Get more of a history ⋯⟩ **057**

> II. Order four units of blood urgently ⋯⟩ **105**

> III. Insert a second IV line ⋯⟩ **053**

> IV. Give more IV fluids ⋯⟩ **011**

015 Cahoon becomes irritated at the argument. He tells you to take another case and to stop wasting his time. **Deduct 1 point**.

⋯⟩ **037**

016 Your hospital does not routinely check serum beta HCG and you must wait for another urine sample which takes another 20 minutes. It returns as positive. **Add 1 point**.

> I. If you want to ask Eileen to tell the mother ⋯⟩ **061**

> II. If you want to tell the girl ⋯⟩ **062**

> III. If you want to tell the mother ⋯⟩ **019**

> IV. If you want to ask Eileen to tell the girl ⋯⟩ **061**

017 The haematologist contacts Cahoon to complain about the potential waste of four precious units of blood. He asks '*What the hell were you playing at, Simpson?*' and looks after the women from here on in. He tells you he will speak to Halsted in the morning. **Deduct 1 point**.

> *I. If you want to argue the case* ⸱⸱⸱⟩ **043**

> *II. If you want to check the slot for more cases* ⸱⸱⸱⟩ **067**

018 The girl agrees to this and you stay while she tells her mother herself. Her mother is shocked but you are surprised how supportive she is. Both seem grateful for your help and you link them up with an obstetrician to perform an ultrasound that confirms the pregnancy and helps with further planning. Pleased with yourself, you walk over to the charts. **Add 2 points**.

> ⸱⸱⸱⟩ **037**

019 The girl starts to cry uncontrollably and Eileen asks you to leave, complaining to her superior that you have upset the patient. Margaret calls in Cahoon who is currently having his supper and explains the situation. He asks '*What the hell were you playing at, Simpson?*' and looks after the girl from here on in. He tells you he will speak to Halsted in the morning. **Deduct 1 point**.

> *I. If you want to argue the case* ⸱⸱⸱⟩ **042**

> *II. If you want to check the slot for more cases* ⸱⸱⸱⟩ **037**

020 Cahoon can't take it any more. He says '*Give me your bleep and go home, I'll get Winston to finish off*'. Your shift is over.

021 Her mother overhears and refuses to allow you to perform a DRE exam, demanding to know what possible reason there is for such a procedure. She has lost all confidence in you and refuses to allow you to treat her daughter. Margaret Hellman, the head nurse, is called over and tries to defuse the situation. She calls in Cahoon who is currently having his supper and explains the situation. He asks '*What the hell were you playing at, Simpson? I'll look after the girl from here on in*'. He tells you he will speak to Halsted in the morning.

> *I. If you want to argue the case* ⸱⸱⸱⟩ **042**

> *II. If you want to check the slot for more cases* ⸱⸱⸱⟩ **037**

022 As you are flicking through the charts in the slot, the girl's mother storms out from behind the curtain and starts to scream at you for leaving her daughter alone in that state. You try to reason but she is hysterical and needs somebody to blame. Margaret Hellman is called over and tries to defuse the situation. She calls Cahoon who is currently having his supper and explains the situation. He asks '*What the hell were you playing at, Simpson?*' and looks after the girl from here on in. He tells you he will speak to Halsted in the morning. **Deduct 1 point**.

> *I. If you want to argue the case* ⋯⧽ **042**
>
> *II. If you want to check the slot for more cases* ⋯⧽ **037**

023 Speaking softly and calmly, you tell her that everything will be fine and that you will find out why she is ill. She looks up at you and with her mother gone, whispers that she has had unprotected sex with her boyfriend several times over the past 3 months. She has not had a period for 8 weeks now. **Add 1 point**.

> *I. If you want to order an immediate pregnancy test* ⋯⧽ **016**
>
> *II. If you want to perform a DRE exam* ⋯⧽ **021**
>
> *III. If you want to tell her that you must bring her mother in and explain* ⋯⧽ **155**
>
> *IV. If you want to leave and check investigations* ⋯⧽ **118**
>
> *V. If you want to leave and order radiology tests* ⋯⧽ **136**

024 **Deduct 1 point**. Will you give a course of antibiotics after draining the abscess?

> *I. Yes* ⋯⧽ **164**
>
> *II. No* ⋯⧽ **027**

025 Pleased with yourself, you begin to flick through the charts again. However, when the girl returns 2 days later with further vomiting, your rival Winston is on call and the first thing he does is order a pregnancy test which is positive. Winston takes great pleasure in sending you a copy. **Deduct 1 point**.

⋯⧽ **037**

026 You administer the diclofenac but the pain diminishes very little and she is still unable to give a history. Furthermore, the NSAID intensifies the damage to her kidneys over the next 2 days and she will require dialysis for renal impairment. **Deduct 1 point**. Margaret is standing beside you and can't believe you're not going to theatre straight away. Do you now:

> *I. Examine her* ⋯⧽ **038**
>
> *II. Order four units of blood urgently* ⋯⧽ **105**
>
> *III. Insert a second IV line* ⋯⧽ **053**

IV. Give more IV fluids ┄┊ 011

V. Get radiology ┄┊ 060

VI. Go to theatre for an exploratory laparotomy ┄┊ 069

027 Antibiotics have no benefit in the immunocompetent patient after the abscess has drained; **add 1 point**. Conscious that Cahoon does not like to sit through unnecessary outpatients, will you:

I. Discharge him ┄┊ 047

II. Bring him back in 3 weeks ┄┊ 082

028 She calls in Cahoon who is currently having his supper and explains the situation. He asks *'What the hell were you playing at, Simpson?'* and looks after the woman from here on in. He tells you he will speak to Halsted in the morning. **Deduct 1 point**.

I. If you want to argue the case ┄┊ 043

II. If you want to check the slot for more cases ┄┊ 067

029 The girl vomits again but settles enough to answer your questions. Her mother becomes agitated that you don't seem to be doing anything, and asks Margaret if there is anybody more senior or older available.

I. If you want to ask the mother to leave the room ┄┊ 154

II. If you want to give her prochlorperazine ┄┊ 003

III. If you want to give her cyclizine ┄┊ 004

IV. If you want to give her ondansetron straight away ┄┊ 079

V. If you want to tell the mother that it is important that you get an idea of what is going on before you treat ┄┊ 065

030 You are wise to try to prioritise; **add 1 point**. The vital signs of all four patients are below:

I. Cellulitis: pulse 76, BP 126/82, Temp 37.7 ┄┊ 110

II. Abdominal pain: pulse 102, BP 90/76, Temp 37.2 ┄┊ 002

031 The ultrasound demonstrates a heartbeat and intrauterine pregnancy. Quickly you realise what you have done by ordering the x-rays without checking her pregnancy status. Margaret calls Cahoon in, who is currently having his supper, and explains the situation. He asks *'What the hell were you playing at, Simpson? Give me your bleep and go home, I'll get Winston to finish your shift and I'll talk to Halsted in the morning'*. Your shift is over.

032 What would you like to give?

   I. Morphine IV ⤏ **049**

   II. Diclofenac PR ⤏ **026**

   III. Paracetamol/acetaminophen PR ⤏ **039**

033 You try talking to the lady but she is too uncomfortable. **Deduct 1 point**. Margaret is standing beside you and still can't believe you're not going to theatre straight away. Will you:

   I. Examine her ⤏ **038**

   II. Administer analgesia ⤏ **032**

   III. Order four units of blood urgently ⤏ **105**

   IV. Insert a second IV line ⤏ **053**

   V. Give more IV fluids ⤏ **011**

   VI. Go to theatre for an exploratory laparotomy ⤏ **069**

034 You start him on his intravenous antibiotics and on the morning ward round Cahoon asks why on earth this man still has a rip-roaring abscess on the side of his neck. '*My God, man, he needs an incision and drainage. Where's Winston?* I'll get him to do it.' **Deduct 1 point**.

⤏ **050**

035 You flick through her chart again, conscious that more surgical charts are mounting up.

   I. If you want to repeat her labs ⤏ **124**

   II. If you want to order a pregnancy test ⤏ **016**

   III. If you want to discharge her with clear instructions to return if her symptoms progress ⤏ **025**

036 The chest x-ray is normal. **Deduct 1 point**.

   I. If you want an ultrasound abdomen ⤏ **031**

   II. If you want a CT abdomen ⤏ **112**

037 There are now two charts in the surgical slot.

   I. To see a 35-year-old man with cellulitis ⤏ **040**

   II. To see a 62-year-old lady with diffuse abdominal pain ⤏ **002**

   III. For more information regarding all cases before you decide ⤏ **030**

038 The lady is diffusely tender with generalised guarding and rebound. Bowel sounds are absent and she is clammy to touch. Her tongue is dry, fissured and cracked.

> *I. Get more of a history* ⋯⟩ **057**

> *II. Administer analgesia* ⋯⟩ **032**

> *III. Order four units of blood urgently* ⋯⟩ **105**

> *IV. Insert a second IV line* ⋯⟩ **053**

> *V. Give more IV fluids* ⋯⟩ **011**

039 Margaret stares at you incredulously as you give PR paracetamol/acetaminophen alone as analgesia for this patient with peritonism and who is crying with pain. Margaret calls in Cahoon, who is currently having his supper, and explains the situation. He asks *'What the hell were you playing at, Simpson?'* and looks after the woman from here on in. He tells you he will speak to Halsted in the morning. **Deduct 1 point**.

> *I. If you want to argue the case* ⋯⟩ **077**

> *II. If you want to check the slot for more cases* ⋯⟩ **067**

040 You pull back the curtain and see a man with a red swollen foot. Just as you are about to introduce yourself, Margaret puts her head around the curtain and asks you to see the lady with epigastric pain. Do you:

> *I. Tell her who the doctor is around here* ⋯⟩ **028**

> *II. Apologise to the gentleman and go and see the other patient* ⋯⟩ **044**

041 The girl stops crying and seems comforted by this. She asks what she will tell her mother and you suggest she could explain everything by saying it was a stomach bug. She hugs you in gratitude and you walk away feeling that you have done a good job. Four weeks from now, Halsted will hear from the girl's mother and her legal representative complaining that her 14-year-old daughter was provided with no follow-up or support. Right now, you feel top of the world and check the charts in your slot. **Deduct 1 point**.

⋯⟩ **037**

042 Cahoon asks how you could have qualified from medical school. He takes your bleep from you and tells you to go home; he will finish the on call on his own. Tomorrow he will speak to Halsted about your behaviour. Your shift is now over.

043 Cahoon asks how you could have qualified from medical school. He takes your bleep from you and tells you to go home; he will finish the on call on his own. Winston can take over tomorrow and he will speak to Halsted about your behaviour. Your shift is over.

044 Sharyn Romanowska is a 62-year-old lady with chronic inflammatory bowel disease, cardiac disease and COPD, who presents with sudden onset of epigastric pain. In her past surgical history she has had a right hemicolectomy and small bowel resection for Crohn's disease more than 10 years ago. Her pulse is 130 and her BP 92/72. Sharyn Romanowska's blood reports can be found in the Investigations at the end of this section. Currently she is sobbing with pain, lying absolutely still on the bed. Margaret is standing beside you and can't believe you're not going to theatre straight away. Do you:

> I. *Examine her* ⋯⋗ **038**

> II. *Get more of a history* ⋯⋗ **033**

> III. *Administer analgesia* ⋯⋗ **032**

> IV. *Order four units of blood urgently* ⋯⋗ **105**

> V. *Insert a second IV line* ⋯⋗ **053**

> VI. *Give more IV fluids* ⋯⋗ **011**

> VII. *Go to theatre for an exploratory laparotomy* ⋯⋗ **069**

045 Do you ask for:

> I. *An ultrasound* ⋯⋗ **129**

> II. *A CT* ⋯⋗ **158**

046 Knowing that a large percentage of laparotomies for penetrating trauma are negative, you decide to keep a close eye on the patient. Over the next 40 minutes he complains of more pain around his abdomen and requires more analgesia. He now has a tachycardia of 124. What will you do?

> I. *Schedule theatre* ⋯⋗ **130**

> II. *Increase the analgesia and continue to observe* ⋯⋗ **131**

047 Two months later Winston is on call and the man returns with another infected sebaceous cyst. Although you performed an incision and drainage, the underlying cyst still remained and has caused further problems. When the man asks why he keeps getting this problem, Winston takes great pleasure in telling him that it is because the first doctor failed to follow up and deal with the cyst. **Deduct 1 point.**

⋯⋗ **050**

048 You try to perform a laparoscopy but there are dense adhesions secondary to her two previous laparotomies and previously active Crohn's disease. You change to an open laparotomy and discover the bile-stained fluid of a perforated duodenum. You close this with an omental patch and the lady is returned to the ICU. Two days later she is transferred from the ICU to the ward and she eventually makes a full recovery. Well done, **add 1 point**. Return to the surgical slot.

⤍ **067**

049 You administer intravenous morphine and the lady's already low blood pressure falls a little but you respond by increasing her fluids.

⤍ **075**

050 You return to the triage slot to find two more charts. Just as you pick them up, a nurse grabs you by the arm, saying 'Hurry, we need you in the resuscitation room'. Your heart quickens as you follow her, feeling important as the people in the department stand out of your way.

⤍ **090**

051 You press firmly around her abdomen but she has no tenderness and no significant findings.

　I. If you want to perform a DRE exam ⤍ **021**

　II. If you want to check her investigations ⤍ **118**

　III. If you want to order radiology tests ⤍ **136**

052 You hang up and decide what to do next.

　I. Examine her ⤍ **106**

　II. Administer analgesia ⤍ **032**

　III. Insert a second IV line ⤍ **053**

　IV. Give more IV fluids ⤍ **011**

　V. Go to theatre for an exploratory laparotomy ⤍ **069**

053 You insert a second IV line to help with your resuscitation. **Add 1 point**. Margaret, the head nurse, still wants to know why this patient hasn't gone to theatre yet. Do you next:

　I. Examine her ⤍ **150**

　II. Administer analgesia ⤍ **032**

　III. Give more IV fluids ⤍ **011**

　IV. Go to theatre for an exploratory laparotomy ⤍ **069**

054 You go and see the girl who now sounds like a priority. You flick quickly through her chart. Karen Twentyman is a 14-year-old girl with no medical history of note. Three days ago she developed mild suprapubic pain with associated nausea and vomiting. The triage nurse has sent off a urine sample for culture. You pull back the curtain and a stocky girl in a school uniform is vomiting into a kidney dish. Her mother rubs her back and looks up as you enter. Eileen, the nurse looking after her, asks you to prescribe an antiemetic in order to make the girl more comfortable.

> I. *If you want to give her prochlorperazine* ⋯⟩ **003**
>
> II. *If you want to give her cyclizine* ⋯⟩ **004**
>
> III. *If you want to give her ondansetron* ⋯⟩ **079**
>
> IV. *If you want to hold off the antiemetics and try to elicit a history first* ⋯⟩ **029**

055 Rightly, you start with a good history. **Add 1 point**. He tells you that his GP put him on co-amoxyclav 3 days ago, but the lump has become more painful. You find a 2 × 2 cm tender, fluctuant mass on the right side of his neck, in keeping with an infected sebaceous cyst.

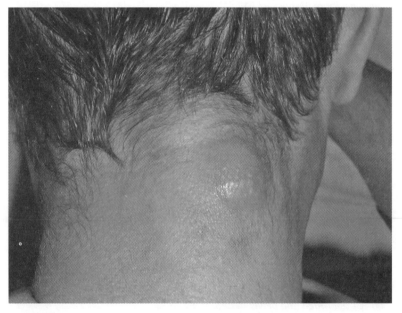

Trent Goeken.

Will you:

> I. *Change him to 500 mg flucloxacillin PO, three times daily* ⋯⟩ **059**
>
> II. *Admit him for IV flucloxacillin and benzylpenicillin* ⋯⟩ **034**
>
> III. *Perform incision and drainage of the abscess* ⋯⟩ **066**

056 You tell Ruth that the girl is tachycardic and peritonitic and will need to go to theatre tonight. Reluctantly she agrees to your request. However, before performing the CT she orders a pregnancy test which is positive. She then examines the patient and realises you have lied. In a fury, she calls Cahoon, who is currently having his supper, and explains the situation. '*What the hell were you playing at, Simpson? Give me your bleep and go home, I'll get Winston to finish your shift and I'll talk to Halsted in the morning,*' he tells you. Your shift is over.

057 You try talking to the lady but she is too uncomfortable. **Deduct 1 point**. Meanwhile Margaret cannot understand why the patient has not gone to theatre yet.

> *I. Administer analgesia* ⋯⟩ **032**

> *II. Order four units of blood urgently* ⋯⟩ **105**

> *III. Insert a second IV line* ⋯⟩ **053**

> *IV. Give more IV fluids* ⋯⟩ **011**

> *V. Go to theatre for an exploratory laparotomy* ⋯⟩ **069**

058 This is exactly what to do. Both Dan's CVP and urine output remain stable since his fluid challenge. You maintain his fluids and he comes down on his inotropes. Well done. **Give yourself 2 points** and

> ⋯⟩ **156.**

059 Pleased with yourself, you discharge the man on oral flucloxacillin. He comes back 2 days later angry that the redness and pain have increased. Winston enjoys performing the incision and drainage of the abscess that should have been performed 2 days earlier. **Deduct 1 point**.

> ⋯⟩ **050**

060 What tests would you like to order?

> *I. Erect chest x-ray* ⋯⟩ **063**

> *II. Plain film of abdomen* ⋯⟩ **068**

> *III. CT abdomen and pelvis* ⋯⟩ **085**

061 The nurse complains to her superior that you are avoiding your responsibilities and that she has her own work to do. Margaret, the head nurse, calls in Cahoon, who is currently having his supper, and explains the situation. He asks '*What the hell were you playing at, Simpson?*' and looks after the girl from here on in. He tells you he will speak to Halsted in the morning. **Deduct 1 point**.

    I. If you want to argue the case ⋯⟫ **042**

    II. If you want to check the slot for more cases ⋯⟫ **037**

062 The girl does not seem surprised and it turns out that she has already used a home tester.

    I. If you want to ask her why the hell she didn't tell you before you considered administering any drugs ⋯⟫ **019**

    II. If you tell her that her mother should know, as she may be able to help ⋯⟫ **155**

    III. If you tell her that she must tell her mother herself ⋯⟫ **019**

    IV. If you want to tell her not to tell her mother and that she has options ⋯⟫ **041**

063 The erect chest x-ray is shown below; **add 1 point**.

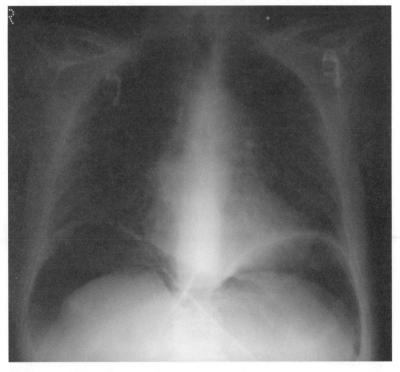

Chest x-ray of Sharyn Romanowska.

Her pain is better controlled and she seems more comfortable. Her pulse is 123, her BP 88/62 and her urine output for the past 1 hour is 16 mL. What do you do next?

    I. Go straight to theatre ⋯⟩ **069**

    II. Get a CT ⋯⟩ **071**

    III. Resuscitate with more fluid ⋯⟩ **078**

064 Rightly, you infiltrate the area around the abscess; **add 1 point**. However, it is still a little uncomfortable. Will you send the pus for culture and sensitivity?

    I. Yes ⋯⟩ **024**

    II. No ⋯⟩ **163**

065 A good history is crucial; **add 1 point**. Karen reports she has felt nausea on and off for a few days with a vague abdominal pain. She only reached menarche earlier this year and her periods have not yet become regular. She denies any drug taking, vaginal symptoms or sexual activity and her bowel function and appetite are normal.

    I. If you want to examine her ⋯⟩ **008**

    II. If you want to look at her investigation results ⋯⟩ **118**

    III. If you want to order radiological tests ⋯⟩ **136**

066 Good job. You are savvy enough to know that it is difficult for antibiotics to penetrate into an abscess, and that this man needs the pus drained. **Add 1 point**. Will you:

    I. Infiltrate the centre of the abscess with local anaesthetic ⋯⟩ **159**

    II. Infiltrate the area around the abscess with local anaesthetic ⋯⟩ **064**

    III. Perform the incision and drainage under general anaesthetic ⋯⟩ **161**

067 There are two cases to see: Undu Ismail, the man with cellulitis, and Trent Goeken, the man with the neck lump. As the man with the cellulitis has been waiting longer, you decide to see him first.

⋯⟩ **080**

068 You request a plain film of abdomen and it adds nothing. **Deduct 1 point** and decide what to do next.

    I. Request an erect chest x-ray ⋯⟩ **063**

    II. Request a CT abdomen ⋯⟩ **085**

069 You waste no time and pressurise Nicola Pablo, the anaesthetist, to put her to sleep for an exploratory laparotomy. Opening her abdomen, you find the bile-stained fluid of a perforated duodenum. Just as you begin to suture an omental patch in place, the lady has a cardiac arrest.

Being profoundly dehydrated and poorly resuscitated before surgery, she is underfilled. This results in increased workload for her already compromised beta-blocked cardiac function. After 30 minutes of cardiac massage, she is declared dead. Cahoon asks how you could have qualified from medical school. He takes your bleep from you and tells you to go home. *'I'll get Winston to finish your shift and I'll talk to Halsted in the morning. Your shift is over.'*

070 The ultrasound demonstrates a heartbeat and intrauterine pregnancy. Embarrassed, and thankful you did not order any radiation, you confirm it with a pregnancy test. The girl does not seem surprised and it turns out that she has already used a home tester.

> I. *If you want to ask her why the hell she didn't tell you before you administered drugs* ⋯⫸ **019**

> II. *If you tell her that her mother should know* ⋯⫸ **155**

> III. *If you tell her that she must tell her mother herself* ⋯⫸ **022**

> IV. *If you want to tell her not to tell her mother and that she has options* ⋯⫸ **041**

071 The CT demonstrates free air and fluid in the peritoneum consistent with a perforation. Although there are reactive changes around the duodenum, Ruth will not commit to whether it is a lower or upper perforation. During the procedure, your poorly resuscitated patient drops her blood pressure and is rushed out of the scanner back to the resuscitation room. **Deduct 1 point**. Her pain is better controlled and she seems more comfortable. Her pulse is 123, her BP 88/62 and her urine output for the past 1 hour is 16 mL. Do you next:

> I. *Go straight to theatre* ⋯⫸ **069**

> II. *Resuscitate with more fluid* ⋯⫸ **078**

072 The CT demonstrates free air and fluid in the peritoneum consistent with a perforation. Although there are reactive changes around the duodenum, Ruth will not commit to whether it is a lower or upper perforation. Do you next:

> I. *Go for laparoscopy* ⋯⫸ **048**

> II. *Go for laparotomy* ⋯⫸ **083**

> III. *Manage conservatively* ⋯⫸ **093**

073 You tell Margaret who the doctor is in this emergency department, asking her not to interfere in your cases again. The conversation is overheard by the mother of the girl, who expresses concern that you are not focused on her daughter. Margaret sympathises and calls in Cahoon, who is having his supper. Irritated at your naivety, he tells you to get another case and he will take over this one. **Deduct 1 point**.

> *I. If you want to argue the case* ⋯⋰ **042**

> *II. If you want to pick a new case* ⋯⋰ **037**

074 Wisely, you remember her previous two laparotomies and Crohn's Disease and you perform a laparotomy. Opening her, you discover the bile-stained fluid of a perforated duodenum. You close this with an omental patch and the lady is returned to the ICU. Well done, **add 3 points**. Return to the surgical slot.

⋯⋰ **067**

075 Within a few minutes the lady settles and tells you that she developed sudden epigastric pain around 40 minutes ago. She has had previous epigastric pain but it has always been milder than this and has been well controlled with omeprazole. Her abdomen is diffusely tender and she is guarding. She is currently taking aspirin, atenolol and steroids. **Add 1 point**. Do you next:

> *I. Get radiology* ⋯⋰ **060**

> *II. Go to theatre for an exploratory laparotomy* ⋯⋰ **069**

076 He is tender maximally over the site of the stab wound with localised guarding but no rebound. Do you next:

> *I. Take a history* ⋯⋰ **113**

> *II. Monitor conservatively* ⋯⋰ **114**

> *III. Schedule theatre* ⋯⋰ **108**

> *IV. Organise imaging* ⋯⋰ **045**

077 Cahoon becomes irritated at the argument. He tells you to take another case and to stop wasting his time. **Deduct 1 point**.

⋯⋰ **067**

078 You administer IV fluids and continue to fluid resuscitate the lady, bringing her urine output up to 32 ml/hour. You also administer antibiotics. Three hours later you are happy that she has been adequately resuscitated. **Add 1 point**. The CT has demonstrated free air and fluid in the peritoneum consistent with a perforation. What would you like to do?

> *I. Laparoscopy* ⋯⋰ **048**

> *II. Laparotomy* ⋯⋰ **083**

> *III. Manage conservatively* ⋯⋰ **093**

079 Margaret grumbles at the expense of wasting drugs like ondansetron when there are cheaper available. **Deduct 1 point.** She tells you she wants to talk to you afterwards in her office. You administer the ondansetron and within a short while Karen settles back. She tells you she has only a dull ache around her belly button. She has no urinary or bowel symptoms and this has never happened before.

> *I. If you want to ask Margaret for a moment and assert your authority early on ⋯⊱* **073**

> *II. If you want to take a further history ⋯⊱* **065**

> *III. If you want to exam her ⋯⊱* **008**

> *IV. If you want to look at her investigation results ⋯⊱* **118**

> *V. If you want to order radiological tests ⋯⊱* **136**

080 You are about to see the man with cellulitis when your intern, Mia, rings in a panic telling you that Jill Baruani, a lady who had varicose veins surgery earlier today, is bleeding from her leg. Her pulse is 92 and her BP is 118/68. Do you:

> *I. Tell Mia to calm down, you'll be there after you have seen this man ⋯⊱* **138**

> *II. Tell her to apply pressure, drop what you're doing and go to the ward ⋯⊱* **006**

081 Concerned about the girl, Margaret rings Cahoon who is now having his supper. Irritated, he tells you to go and see the girl. Margaret smiles smugly as you apologise to the man with the cellulitis and go to the girl. **Deduct 1 point.**

⋯⊱ **054**

082 Well done for realising that although sometimes the infection can destroy the cyst, equally it may persist and cause further problems. Following him up in the OPD allows you to examine him and if necessary excise the cyst. **Add 2 points.**

⋯⊱ **050**

083 Wisely, you remember her previous two laparotomies and Crohn's Disease and you perform a laparotomy. Opening her, you discover the bile-stained fluid of a perforated duodenum. You close this with an omental patch and the lady is returned to the ICU. Two days later she is transferred from the ICU to the ward and she eventually makes a full recovery. Well done, **add 3 points.** Return to the surgical slot.

⋯⊱ **067**

084 Cahoon comes to the ward within a few minutes. He examines the leg and observes that the bleed is obviously venous. He applies a small wedge of folded gauze to the area and wraps a compression dressing around it. This stops the bleeding. He puts his jacket back on and tells you he'll see you in the morning but if there are any more problems overnight to ring him.

⋯⟶ **137**

085 Ruth insists on a portable erect chest x-ray first, given the fact that the lady has been unstable and is not yet fully resuscitated. **Deduct 1 point**.

⋯⟶ **063**

086 You rightly raise the leg in the air to reduce venous flow and compress the bleeding point. Conscious that it may start again later, you wrap the leg with a compression dressing and the bleeding stops. Mia smiles in gratitude. Happy with yourself, you return to the emergency department. **Give yourself 2 points**.

⋯⟶ **137**

087 In order to reduce the chance of missing important information, you should always start with a history; **deduct 1 point**. He tells you that his GP put him on co-amoxyclav 3 days ago, but the lump has become more painful. You find a 2 × 2 cm tender, fluctuant mass on the right side of his neck, in keeping with an infected sebaceous cyst.

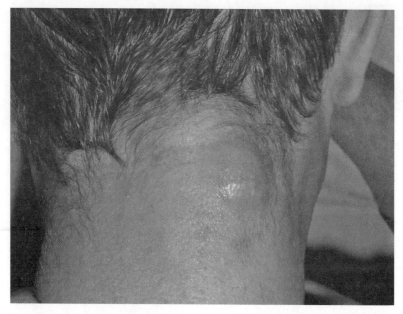

Trent Goeken.

Will you:

> I. *Change him to 500 mg flucloxacillin PO, three times daily* ⋯⟶ **059**

> II. *Admit him for IV flucloxacillin and benzylpenicillin* ⋯⟶ **034**

> III. *Perform incision and drainage of the abscess* ⋯⟶ **066**

088 The chest x-ray is normal, **deduct 1 point**.

> I. *If you want a plain film of abdomen* ⋯⟶ **151**

> II. *If you want an ultrasound abdomen* ⋯⟶ **031**

> III. *If you want a CT abdomen* ⋯⟶ **112**

089 You can do better. It sounds like you may have missed finishing some of the cases. You managed to keep your score in positive figures which is good. Review the Perspectives section and see if you can build on this in the next section.

090 Grabbing a pair of gloves, you push through the doors of the resus room and see a young man being transferred onto a trolley holding his abdomen. The paramedic looks up, relieved to see you. '*David Cummins, 21 year old male found on the street 20 minutes ago with a single stab wound to his central abdomen. Minimal blood loss, pulse 106, BP 130/84, O₂ sats 98% on 100% oxygen.*' The man is curled over and has his hands pressed under his umbilicus. What do you do next?

> I. *Start taking a history, assessing if he can speak* ⋯⟶ **132**

> II. *Get a better look at his abdomen* ⋯⟶ **100**

> III. *Put in a urinary catheter* ⋯⟶ **146**

> IV. *Put in an intravenous line* ⋯⟶ **102**

> V. *Get central line access* ⋯⟶ **098**

091 The lady is diffusely tender with generalised guarding and rebound. Bowel sounds are absent and she is clammy to touch. Her tongue is dry, fissured and cracked. Do you want to:

> I. *Get more of a history* ⋯⟶ **057**

> II. *Administer analgesia* ⋯⟶ **032**

> III. *Order four units of blood urgently* ⋯⟶ **105**

> IV. *Insert a second IV line* ⋯⟶ **053**

> V. *Give more IV fluids* ⋯⟶ **011**

092 You pull back the curtain and see a 35-year old-man with a red inflamed foot. As you start, a nurse puts her head around the curtain and tells you that the girl is vomiting again. Do you:

I. Continue with your current patient ⋯⃗ **081**

II. Go and see the girl ⋯⃗ **054**

093 Although the lady has responded to your resuscitation efforts, she is peritonitic. Over the next 24 hours her renal function continues to deteriorate and she becomes septic. **Deduct 1 point**. What will you do now?

I. Laparoscopy ⋯⃗ **009**

II. Laparotomy ⋯⃗ **074**

094 You can do better. Sometimes it is not enough to know just the theory. How to handle people and situations is as crucial in medicine as knowing the facts and figures. The only way to improve on this is experience. Review the Perspectives at the end of this section and, using what you have learned, try the next section. See if you can build on this.

095 The haematologist on call becomes irate at your flippant attitude towards blood. *'You know this man's Hb is 14.2 and there is no evidence he is bleeding, and you want to transfuse him?'* **Deduct 1 point**.

⋯⃗ **153**

096 Excellent. You have demonstrated a fine combination of both knowledge and situation management. It is not enough to have one and not the other. Of course, there is more than one way to manage a situation. It is clear that you chose wisely; however, just because others handle a problem differently does not necessarily mean they handle it incorrectly. Try again and experiment with different styles. Review the Perspectives section and see if you can build on this in the next section for your overall score.

097 **Add 1 point**. The patient has a pulse of 110, BP 90/54, temp 37.2 and a respiratory rate of 18. His CVP measures 4 and was 12 immediately postoperatively. His urine output for the last hour is 12 ml. His abdomen is not distended and mildly tender in keeping with postoperative findings. Do you:

I. Check his blood results ⋯⃗ **149**

II. Transfuse him ⋯⃗ **101**

III. Give him IV fluids ⋯⃗ **122**

098 You are scrubbing up to insert the central line when one of the senior emergency doctors passes and asks what you're doing. When he sees the patient, he takes over: *'Looks like you're starting out, kid, and this guy needs a few things done before we start sticking needles in his neck. I'll look after it from here'*. He completes the ABCs and stabilises the patient. After a CT, he calls Cahoon and David is taken to theatre.

⋯⋗ **134**

099 You try talking to the lady but she is still too sore to talk. Margaret is anxious that the patient goes to theatre as soon as possible. Do you:

   I. Administer morphine ⋯⋗ **075**

   II. Get radiology ⋯⋗ **060**

   III. Go to theatre for an exploratory laparotomy ⋯⋗ **069**

100 The man pushes your hand away as you try to examine him. Persisting, you manage to see a 1 cm wound under his umbilicus. There is no active bleeding and he is tender around the stab area with localised tenderness but no rebound. What will you do next?

   I. Contact Nicola Pablo and schedule theatre ⋯⋗ **109**

   II. Monitor over the next hour ⋯⋗ **144**

   III. Try to take a history ⋯⋗ **127**

101 The haematologist on call becomes irate at your flippant attitude towards blood. *'Have you not bothered to check this man's Hb? There is no evidence he is bleeding, and you want to transfuse him?'* **Deduct 1 point**.

⋯⋗ **152**

102 You quickly insert a large-bore cannula. Caroline, the nurse helping you, asks if you should not assess the ABCs and examine his abdomen. Embarrassed, you agree. **Deduct 1 point** for ignoring the ABCs and losing the confidence of your colleagues.

   I. Start taking a history ⋯⋗ **128**

   II. Get a better look at his abdomen ⋯⋗ **100**

103 The man calms down a little and allows you to examine his abdomen. He has a small 1 cm wound to his infraumbilical area and is tender over the area with localised guarding but no rebound. Jill, the nurse helping you, notices that the patient is gasping for breath. She quickly draws your attention to the patient's low O_2 saturations of 78%. Examining his thorax, you see he has bruising over his lower left ribs with a palpable fracture. Chest x-ray reveals a large pneumothorax on the left side. Certainly this is something you did not want to miss and you should have started your assessment with the ABCs of trauma. **Deduct 1 point** from your score for wasting time. You finish your ABCs and notice that the man has free air under his diaphragm. He is tender with localised guarding around his wound site. Do you:

> *I. Schedule theatre* ⋯⟩ **108**

> *II. Monitor conservatively* ⋯⟩ **046**

> *III. Order a CT* ⋯⟩ **158**

104 You quickly insert a large-bore cannula. Jill, the nurse helping you, notices that the patient is gasping for breath. She quickly draws your attention to the patient's low O_2 saturations of 78%. Examining his thorax, you see he has bruising over his lower left ribs with a palpable fracture. Chest x-ray reveals a large pneumothorax on the left side. Certainly this is something you did not want to miss and you should have started your assessment with the ABCs of trauma. **Deduct 1 point** from your score for wasting time. You finish your ABCs and notice that the man has free air under his diaphragm. Do you:

> *I. Examine his abdomen* ⋯⟩ **076**

> *II. Schedule theatre* ⋯⟩ **108**

105 You try ordering blood from the blood bank but they are reluctant to make the blood available as they argue that her Hb is 15. Do you

> *I. Insist you are the doctor and she needs the blood* ⋯⟩ **017**

> *II. Ask if they can simply group and hold her information for the time being* ⋯⟩ **052**

106 The lady is diffusely tender with generalised guarding and rebound. Bowel sounds are absent and she is clammy to touch. Her tongue is dry, fissured and cracked.

> *I. Get more of a history* ⋯⟩ **057**

> *II. Administer analgesia* ⋯⟩ **032**

> *III. Insert a second IV line* ⋯⟩ **053**

> *IV. Give more IV fluids* ⋯⟩ **011**

107 His peripheries are warm, his pulse is 102 and his BP is 148/90. You insert two wide-bore cannulae, send bloods and administer analgesia. After the analgesia, the man calms down a little and his pulse falls to 86. **Add 1 point.** Just below his umbilicus is a tangential wound about 1 cm wide. There is no active bleeding at the site. Do you:

   I. Schedule theatre ⋯⟶ **109**

   II. Palpate his abdomen ⋯⟶ **162**

   III. Monitor him conservatively ⋯⟶ **046**

   IV. Organise imaging ⋯⟶ **045**

   V. Get an erect chest x-ray ⋯⟶ **119**

108 Will you perform a:

   I. Laparotomy ⋯⟶ **147**

   II. Laparoscopy ⋯⟶ **142**

109 You call Nicola and she agrees to arrange surgery. Thirty minutes later Nicola storms through the department, furiously waving an x-ray. '*What the hell are you playing at?*' she demands. The rest of the department stops to listen. '*This man was kicked about before he was stabbed and has bruising across his thorax. This is the large pneumothorax you missed. You would have had me put a tube down this man's throat with this! I'm ringing Halsted.*' You try to reason with her but she has a foul temper. Right there in the department in front of everyone, she rings Cahoon. Shouting at Cahoon down the phone, she hands it to you and walks off. Timidly you take the phone. '*What the hell are you doing?*' Cahoon asks. Before you can start, he continues, '*Just go home and I'll get Winston to finish tonight. I can't be worrying all night about what you're going to do, we'll talk about this tomorrow*'. Putting the phone down, you gather your stuff with Margaret the head nurse watching. '*Never mind, kid, maybe this kind of work isn't for you*', she says before walking away.

110 Your priorities are all wrong. Obviously the lady with the abdominal pain is worst and should be seen first. **Deduct 1 point**.

⋯⟶ **044**

111 You get another chart while the nurses monitor the young man's condition over the next hour. About 40 minutes later, the nurse looking after him rushes out to say that he has dropped his oxygen saturations and is gasping for breath. Running in, you find him bent over and pale with a O_2 saturation of 78% and a pulse of 156. Quickly, you listen to his lungs and he has no breath sounds on the left-hand side. The chest x-ray which was performed as part of the trauma series demonstrates a pneumothorax on the left side. You quickly insert a chest drain and the patient slowly improves. However, Jill, the nurse looking after the patient, has some serious concerns and contacts the head nurse Margaret. Margaret rings Cahoon, who storms into the department demanding to know why you didn't examine the patient properly. Your excuses fall on deaf ears and he sends you home: *'I can't work with you, you're dangerous, and I'm getting Winston in to cover'*. You leave the resus room as Margaret walks away. Your shift is over.

112 Ruth Benedict, your radiologist, argues that a CT is not indicated in a girl of 14 with *soft* signs due to the risk from radiation.

> *I. If you want to argue further, exaggerating the findings on exam in order to get the test done* ⋯⟩ **056**

> *II. If you want to back down and rethink* ⋯⟩ **035**

113 The man tells you that he was robbed and his attacker stabbed him with a screwdriver. He suffered no other injury but his belly hurts. You complete your secondary survey and can find no other injuries. Do you next:

> *I. Monitor him conservatively* ⋯⟩ **046**

> *II. Schedule theatre* ⋯⟩ **117**

> *III. Organise a CT* ⋯⟩ **135**

> *IV. Get an erect chest x-ray* ⋯⟩ **121**

114 Over the next hour his pain increases with a tachycardia of 128 and a BP 156/90. Margaret becomes increasingly anxious about his condition.

> *I. Schedule theatre* ⋯⟩ **108**

> *II. Increase the analgesia and continue to observe* ⋯⟩ **131**

115 Karen seems pleased that you are getting a nurse. It takes you 10 minutes to find a free nurse to chaperone you; **add 1 point**. Her mother leaves as the nurse arrives and she waits outside the curtains. You press firmly around the girl's abdomen but she has no tenderness and no significant findings. She starts to cry.

> *I. If you want to wait before continuing your examination* ⋯⟩ **023**

> *II. If you want to complete your examination quickly with a rectal examination in order to minimise her distress* ⋯⟩ **021**

116 Rightly, you continue assessing the ABCs and listen to the man's lungs. He has equal breath sounds, there is no tracheal shift, his respiratory rate is 15 and his oxygen saturation is 99%. **Add 1 point**. What will you do next?

> *I. Examine his abdomen* ⋯⟩ **162**

> *II. Assess his circulation* ⋯⟩ **107**

> *III. Schedule theatre* ⋯⟩ **108**

IV. Organise a CT ⤍ **135**

V. Get an erect chest x-ray ⤍ **119**

117 The man has signs of peritonism and you are obliged to investigate further. Although a CT or chest x-ray may demonstrate free air or fluid, with peritonism you are still committed to surgery. Will you:

I. Perform a laparotomy ⤍ **147**

II. Perform a laparoscopy ⤍ **142**

118 Karen Twentyman's bloods are found in the Investigation section at the end of the book.

I. If you want to order radiology tests ⤍ **136**

II. If you want to repeat her labs ⤍ **124**

III. If you want order a pregnancy test ⤍ **016**

IV. If you want to discharge with clear instructions to return if her symptoms progress ⤍ **025**

119 The chest x-ray demonstrates normal lungs but a small amount of free air under the right diaphragm. He is tender maximally over the site of the stab wound with localised guarding but no rebound.

I. Manage him conservatively ⤍ **114**

II. Schedule theatre ⤍ **108**

120 By the time the morning comes around he is tachycardic and his urine output is only 8 mL for the last hour. He required more fluids overnight and Cahoon is not impressed. Winston grins at your discomfort.

⤍ **156**

121 Chest x-ray reveals a large pneumothorax on the left side. Certainly this is something you did not want to miss and you should have started your assessment with the ABCs of trauma. **Deduct 1 point** from your score. You finish your ABCs and notice that the man has free air under his diaphragm. Do you:

I. Watch conservatively ⤍ **114**

II. Schedule theatre ⤍ **108**

122 Good decision. The man's output is reduced, his CVP is down, his urine specific gravity is increased, his HCT is increased and his urea is increased with a normal creatinine. The picture is that of dehydration. You give him a fluid challenge of 500 ml over 30 minutes and his pulse slows to 88, BP rises to 134/76, urine climbs to 30 ml and CVP rises to 6. **Give yourself 1 point**. Do you:

> *I. Recheck his fluid status in one hour* ⋯⟩ **058**

> *II. Check again in the morning* ⋯⟩ **120**

123 Mia tells you that Dan Schoenberger is a 54-year-old, 60 kg man who is post anterior resection by about 4 hours. The procedure was unusually long as his lesion was quite low down and he had a difficult narrow pelvis. However, blood loss was minimal and the team were happy with the result. He was returned to the unit as he was a little drowsy post intubation. You go to the ICU and, taking a history, he tells you he is comfortable. However, his blood pressure is low at 90/54. The anaesthetic junior doctor has commenced a noradrenaline infusion to improve it, but his response has been slow. Do you:

> *I. Leave it in the hands of the anaesthetist* ⋯⟩ **143**

> *II. Examine him* ⋯⟩ **097**

> *III. Check his blood results* ⋯⟩ **145**

> *IV. Transfuse him* ⋯⟩ **101**

> *V. Give him IV fluids* ⋯⟩ **122**

124 The girl's repeat labs and urine are normal and her mother is getting impatient.

> *I. If you want to order a pregnancy test* ⋯⟩ **016**

> *II. If you want to discharge with clear instructions to return if her symptoms progress* ⋯⟩ **025**

125 The CT demonstrates free air and fluid in the peritoneum consistent with a perforation. Although there are reactive changes around the duodenum, Ruth will not commit to whether it is a lower or upper perforation. Do you next:

> *I. Go straight to theatre* ⋯⟩ **069**

> *II. Resuscitate with more fluid* ⋯⟩ **078**

126 You get another chart while the nurses monitor the young man's condition over the next hour. About 40 minutes later, the nurse looking after him rushes out to say that he has dropped his oxygen saturations and is gasping for breath. Running in, you find him bent over and pale with a O_2 saturation of 78% and a pulse of 156. Quickly, you listen to his lungs and he has no breath sounds on the left-hand side. The chest x-ray which was performed as part of the trauma series demonstrates a pneumothorax on the left side. You quickly insert a chest drain and the patient slowly improves. However Izzy, the nurse looking after the patient, has some serious concerns and contacts the head nurse Margaret. Margaret rings Cahoon, who storms into the department demanding to know why you didn't examine the patient properly. Your excuses fall on deaf ears and he sends you home: '*I can't work with you, you're dangerous, and I'm getting Winston in to cover*'. You leave the resus room as Margaret walks away. Your shift is over.

127 Taking a history, the patient tells you that he was badly kicked about the chest before being stabbed. Examining his thorax, you see he has bruising over his lower left ribs with a palpable fracture. Chest x-ray reveals a large pneumothorax on the left side. Certainly, this is something you did not want to miss and you should have started your assessment with the ABCs of trauma. **Deduct 1 point** from your score. You finish your ABCs and notice that the man has free air under his diaphragm. Do you:

> I. *Examine his abdomen* ⋯⟩ **076**

> II. *Insert a chest drain and schedule theatre* ⋯⟩ **108**

128 By starting to talk to the man, you have prioritised assessment of his airway. You ask him what happened and he looks up and curses at you. Relieved that he can obviously maintain his own airway, do you next:

> I. *Tell him you are trying to help and examine his abdomen* ⋯⟩ **103**

> II. *Get peripheral intravenous access* ⋯⟩ **104**

> III. *Get central line access* ⋯⟩ **098**

> IV. *Listen to his lungs* ⋯⟩ **116**

129 The ultrasound is reported as normal. What will you do next?

> I. *Organise a CT* ⋯⟩ **158**

> II. *Schedule theatre* ⋯⟩ **108**

> III. *Watch conservatively* ⋯⟩ **046**

130 Will you perform a:

> I. *Laparotomy* ⋯⟩ **147**

> II. *Laparoscopy* ⋯⟩ **142**

131 You get another chart while Izzy watches your patient in resus. The extra morphine seems to have helped, and he is sedated. However, Izzy must take lunch and another nurse covers while she is gone. Distracted by a demented geriatric patient, she does not notice that your patient has now a heart rate of 150 and a temperature of 40°C. Margaret sees what has happened and sends the nurse away. Next she rings Cahoon who storms into the department demanding to know why you didn't watch your patient properly. You try to reason with him but he is not listening. The patient has a perforated sigmoid colon, with faecal peritonitis. He requires a resection and a defunctioning colostomy. Your excuses fall on deaf ears and Cahoon sends you home: *'I can't work with you, you're dangerous, and I'm getting Winston in to cover'.* You leave the resus room as Margaret walks away. Your shift is over.

132 This is exactly the thing to do; **add 1 point**. By starting to talk to the man, you have prioritised assessment of his airway. You ask him what happened and he looks up and curses at you. Relieved that he can obviously maintain his own airway, do you next:

> *I. Tell him you are trying to help and examine his abdomen* ⋯⟩ **103**

> *II. Get peripheral intravenous access* ⋯⟩ **104**

> *III. Get central line access* ⋯⟩ **098**

> *IV. Listen to his lungs* ⋯⟩ **116**

133 Not bad. You managed to negotiate around some difficult situations. The key to improving on this is experience. The doctors that seem good at this are not born that way; it is simply a matter of experience. Review the case Perspectives and see if you can build on this in the next section.

134 You return to the slot but your intern, Mia, calls again.

⋯⟩ **140**

135 You send him for a CT and return to the computer to check some bloods. About 10 minutes later you hear the arrest team bleep go off from the radiology department. Racing down, you find the team performing chest compressions on your patient and squeezing in fluid through an intravenous line. Ruth has rung Cahoon, who comes bursting through the door. *'What the hell is happening here?'* he demands. Quickly assessing the patient, who now has a pulse again but is hypotensive, he rings theatre and tells them he is on the way. Pushing past you, he tells you to *'get the hell out of my sight. What were you thinking, sending an unstable patient to the CT scanner?'.* You're left alone in the room as everyone else rushes off with your patient. Your shift is over.

136 You ring Ruth.

> *I. If you want a chest x-ray* ⋯⟩ **088**

> *II. If you want a plain film of abdomen* ⋯⟩ **007**

III. If you want an ultrasound abdomen ⋯⟩ **070**

IV. If you want a CT abdomen ⋯⟩ **112**

137 You go to see the man with the cellulitis but he has gone outside for a cigarette. You go and see the other patient while you are waiting. He is a 17-year-old man named Trent Goeken who has had a painful lump on the back of his neck for 6 days. Will you:

I. Examine ⋯⟩ **087**

II. Take a history ⋯⟩ **055**

138 Not knowing what to do, Mia calls Cahoon who immediately rushes to the ward. You are in the middle of seeing the man with cellulitis when he bursts in. *'What the hell did you think you were doing?'* He gives you a dressing down in front of everyone for failing to attend the patient who should have been your priority, as well as abandoning a junior colleague. He tells you that if he has anything to do with it, you'll be off call from tomorrow. The stare of every patient and staff member in the department bores a hole through the back of your head as Cahoon takes your bleep and sends you home. Winston's going to love hearing about this in the morning.

139 Mia holds the leg up and dabs the blood away while, after local anaesthetic, you put a small stitch in the oozing point, stopping the bleeding. Mia smiles sweetly in gratitude. Happy with yourself, you return to the emergency department.

⋯⟩ **137**

140 Mia, your intern, is concerned about a postoperative patient in the ICU. Do you:

I. Go to the ICU ⋯⟩ **160**

II. Look for more information ⋯⟩ **123**

141 You contact Nicola and she agrees to arrange surgery. Thirty minutes later Nicola storms through the department, furiously waving an x-ray. *'What the hell are you playing at?'* she demands. The rest of the department stops to listen. *'This man was kicked about before he was stabbed and has bruising across his thorax. This is the large pneumothorax you missed. You would have had me put a tube down this man's throat with this! I'm ringing Halsted.'* You try to reason with her but she has a foul temper. Right there in the department, in front of everyone, she rings Cahoon. Shouting at Cahoon down the phone, she hands it to you and walks off. Timidly you take the phone. *'What the hell are you doing?'* Cahoon asks. Before you can start, he continues, *'Just go home and I'll get Winston to finish tonight. I can't be worrying all night about what you're going to do, we'll talk about this tomorrow'*. Putting the phone down, you gather your stuff with Margaret, the head nurse, watching. *'Never mind, kid, maybe this kind of work isn't for you'*, she says before walking away.

142 You contact Cahoon and tell him your plans. He agrees completely and is very impressed with how you handled the case. Upon laparoscopy, there is a laceration to the omentum and some old blood in the peritoneum. You can see no active bleeding and the bowel is undamaged. *Give yourself 2 points* and prepare to see your next patient.

⋯⋗ **134**

143 The following morning Cahoon castigates you for missing the fact that your patient was dehydrated and was on inotropes unnecessarily. **Deduct 1 point**.

⋯⋗ **156**

144 You get another chart while Izzy watches your patient in resus. The extra morphine seems to have helped, and he is sedated. However, Izzy must take lunch and another nurse covers while she is gone. Distracted by a demented geriatric patient, she does not notice that your patient has a respiratory rate of 38 and an oxygen saturation of 78%. Margaret sees what has happened and calls Cahoon, who storms into the department demanding to know why you didn't watch your patient properly. You try to reason with him but he is not listening. The patient has a pneumothorax that should have been spotted. Your excuses fall on deaf ears and he sends you home: *'I can't work with you, you're dangerous, and I'm getting Winston in to cover'*. You leave the resus room as Margaret walks away. Your shift is over.

145 Bloods sent by Mia 20 minutes ago on Dan Schoenberger can be found in the Investigations at the end of this section. Do you:

I. Leave it in the hands of the anaesthetist ⋯⋗ **143**

II. Examine him ⋯⋗ **097**

III. Transfuse him ⋯⋗ **101**

IV. Give him IV fluids ⋯⋗ **122**

146 You prepare a urinary catheter set in order to monitor his hourly output. Izzy, the nurse helping you, asks if you should not assess his ABCs and examine his abdomen first before doing this. Embarrassed, you say *'Definitely, I was just about to do that'*. **Deduct 1 point** for ignoring the ABCs and losing the confidence of your colleagues.

I. Start taking a history ⋯⟩ **128**

II. Get a better look at his abdomen ⋯⟩ **100**

147 You contact Cahoon and tell him your plans. He agrees that this man certainly needs surgery but he feels that it is worth looking with a laparoscope first. Upon laparoscopy, there is a laceration to the omentum and some old blood in the peritoneum. You can see no active bleeding and the bowel is undamaged. **Give yourself 1 point** and prepare for your next patient.

⋯⟩ **134**

148 You pull a tourniquet tightly just proximal to the bleeding point. Jill Baruani screams as it tightens. Caroline, the staff nurse with Jill, looks on nervously and comments that she has never seen a tourniquet being used in this way before. You ring Cahoon, waking him, and explain what has happened. He shouts at you to take the tourniquet off, elevate the leg and apply some pressure. He tells you he's on his way in. Fifteen minutes later, he arrives on the ward and tells you to take your hand away. The bleeding has now stopped and he wraps a second compression bandage around the leg, *'We'll talk about bleeding in the morning, Simpson,'* he says, putting on his jacket. Turning to Caroline, he mutters *'If genius here has any more of these bright ideas, ring me first'*. Embarassed in front of your intern and the staff nurse, you return to the emergency department. **Deduct 1 point**.

⋯⟩ **137**

149 Bloods sent by your intern 20 minutes ago on Dan Schoenberger can be found in the Investigations at the end of this section. **Add 1 point**. Do you:

I. Leave it in the hands of the anaesthetist ⋯⟩ **143**

II. Transfuse him ⋯⟩ **095**

III. Give him IV fluids ⋯⟩ **122**

150 The lady is diffusely tender with generalised guarding and rebound. Bowel sounds are absent and she is clammy to touch. Her tongue is dry, fissured and cracked.

I. Get more of a history ⋯⟩ **057**

II. Administer analgesia ⋯⟩ **032**

III. Order four units of blood urgently ⋯⟩ **105**

IV. Give more IV fluids ⋯⟩ **011**

151 The plain film of abdomen is normal. **Deduct 1 point**.

I. If you want an ultrasound abdomen ⋯⟩ **070**

II. If you want a CT abdomen ⋯⟩ **112**

152 Bloods sent by your intern 20 minutes ago on Dan Schoenberger can be found in the Investigations at the end of this section. Do you:

I. *Leave it in the hands of the anaesthetist* ⇢ **143**

II. *Give him IV fluids* ⇢ **122**

153 Do you:

I. *Leave it in the hands of the anaesthetist* ⇢ **143**

II. *Give him IV fluids* ⇢ **005**

154 Her mother refuses to leave her daughter without a chaperone. She becomes annoyed at your flippant attitude. She has lost all confidence in you and refuses to allow you treat her daughter. Margaret is called over and tries to defuse the situation. She calls Cahoon, who is forced to stop operating to take the call. He asks '*What the hell were you playing at, Simpson? I'll have to leave theatre and look after the girl from here on in*'. You explain that the mother is very anxious and has been difficult to deal with. Cahoon calms a little but tells you that you should have handled it better. In the background, you hear Halsted demanding to know what is going on.

I. *If you want to argue the case* ⇢ **042**

II. *If you want to check the slot for more cases* ⇢ **037**

155 The girl begs you not to tell her mother.

I. *If you want to offer to stay while she tells her mother* ⇢ **018**

II. *If you want to suggest she tells her mother on her own* ⇢ **022**

III. *If you want to tell her not to tell her mother and that she has options* ⇢ **041**

156 You return to the emergency department but your man with cellulitis still has not come back to his bed, and another patient has decided to go home. The surgical slot is empty and you take your opportunity to grab a quick break while the medical team see their fifth collapse of unknown cause. ⇢ **157** to calculate your points.

157 Add up your points.

I. *If you scored a negative figure* ⇢ **094**

II. *If you scored between 1 and 16* ⇢ **089**

III. *If you scored between 17 and 33* ⇢ **133**

IV. *If you scored >34* ⇢ **096**

158 The CT scan demonstrates a small amount of free air and free fluid in his pelvis. There is no extravasation of contrast. Will you:

> I. Schedule theatre ⋯⟩ **108**

> II. Watch conservatively ⋯⟩ **046**

159 The local anaesthetic is ineffective and Mr Goeken suffers a considerable degree of pain during the procedure; **deduct 1 point**. Will you send the pus for culture and sensitivity?

> I. Yes ⋯⟩ **024**

> II. No ⋯⟩ **163**

160 Arriving in the ICU, Mia fills you in on the details. Dan Schoenberger is a 54-year-old man who is post anterior resection by about 4 hours. The procedure was unusually long as his lesion was quite low down and he had a difficult narrow pelvis. However, blood loss was minimal and the team were happy with the result. He was returned to the unit as he was a little drowsy post intubation. Taking a history, he tells you he is comfortable. However, his blood pressure is low at 90/54. The anaesthetic junior doctor has commenced a noradrenaline infusion to improve it but his response has been slow. Do you:

> I. Leave it in the hands of the anaesthetist ⋯⟩ **143**

> II. Examine him ⋯⟩ **097**

> III. Check his blood results ⋯⟩ **145**

> IV. Transfuse him ⋯⟩ **101**

> V. Give him IV fluids ⋯⟩ **005**

161 You bring him to theatre and incise and drain the abscess under general anaesthetic. The bed manager is not impressed that he must find an extra bed tonight as he is having to stay late to do it. However, the patient is very comfortable and goes home the following morning. Will you send the pus for culture and sensitivity?

> I. Yes ⋯⟩ **024**

> II. No ⋯⟩ **163**

162 He is tender maximally over the site of the stab wound with localised guarding but no rebound. Do you next:

> I. Take a history ⋯⟩ **113**

> II. Monitor conservatively ⋯⟩ **114**

> III. Schedule theatre ⋯⟩ **108**

IV. Organise imaging ⤏ 045

V. Get an erect chest x-ray ⤏ 119

163 Well done; culturing the pus does not influence your management of the patient. **Add 1 point**. Will you give a course of antibiotics after draining the abscess?

I. Yes ⤏ 164

II. No ⤏ 027

164 **Deduct 1 point**. Conscious that Cahoon does not like to sit through unnecessary outpatients, will you:

I. Discharge him ⤏ 047

II. Bring him back in 3 weeks ⤏ 082

165 While there is no indication of bleeding currently, it would certainly be prudent to group and save her serum. Next, do you:

I. Examine her ⤏ 038

II. Get more of a history ⤏ 033

III. Administer analgesia ⤏ 032

IV. Insert a second IV line ⤏ 053

V. Give more IV fluids ⤏ 011

VI. Go to theatre for an exploratory laparotomy ⤏ 069

PERSPECTIVES

Case perspectives: Karen Twentyman

THERAPEUTIC PERSPECTIVES

1 Nausea and vomiting in pregnancy

- Eighty percent of women will experience nausea or vomiting in pregnancy, with 52% experiencing both nausea and vomiting. The mean time to onset has been shown to be 39 days, with mean time to resolution 84 days.[1]
- Prochlorperazine has been used to treat nausea and vomiting in pregnancy. It does cross the placenta but the majority of evidence appears to suggest that it is not teratogenic,* despite anecdotal reports of malformations.[2]
- Cyclizine is a H1 receptor antagonist (antihistamine). This group of drugs has been reported to be safe in pregnancy. Whether because of decreasing the metabolic upset or through some other factor, there has been a suggestion that this family of drugs demonstrated a slight reduction in congenital malformations.[3]
- Ondansetron may be safe, and certainly animal studies[4] and some limited human studies have not demonstrated it to be teratogenic.[5] However, it has not been extensively evaluated in the human setting, and as such currently is not considered first line.[6]
- Of the drugs examined in a recent Cochrane review of nausea and vomiting in pregnancy, pyridoxine (vitamin B6) was considered the least likely to cause side-effects.[6]

KAREN AND PRESCRIBING

It is clear that Karen benefitted from an antiemetic and from the evidence presented above, it would appear that her baby is unlikely to suffer because of the use of antiemetics. However, the approach of prescribing blindly should not be encouraged. Had you waited for more information before prescribing, you would have been awarded points. Furthermore, given that there is insufficient evidence to support ondansetron as first-line treatment, if you chose this option you were deducted points. Note: apart from a positive beta HCG, the only other notable abnormality on Karen's investigations is that her urine is positive for ketones. This is as a result of her vomiting; however, clearly she is hydrated enough as she shows no other signs of biochemical dehydration.

*please refer to the Definitions at the end of this Case perspective.

2 Chaperones

- The American Academy of Pediatrics recommends that[7]:
  - the purpose and scope of the physical examination should be made clear to parents
  - it should also be made clear to the patient if he or she is old enough to understand
  - if any part of the examination will be physically or psychologically uncomfortable, the parents and patients should be informed in advance of the examination
  - regarding a chaperone, the highest priority must be given to the requests of the patient and the parents.
- Sixty percent of male doctors use chaperones for medicolegal reasons, while 59% of female doctors use chaperones for technical assistance.[8]
- Most medical defence organisations recommend the use of a chaperone when examining members of the opposite sex.
- One study has demonstrated that 46% of teenage girls prefer a chaperone to be present during a breast, pelvic or rectal examination by a male physician.[9]

KAREN AND EXAMINING

It is clear in this case that Karen's mother wanted a chaperone to be present. Although emotional and anxious, Karen herself appears relieved when you look for a nurse as a chaperone. As laid out in the American Academy of Pediatrics position statement, highest priority must be given to the requests of the patient and the parents. In this case both parent and patient appear to want a chaperone. Failing to recognise this in what is an emotionally charged atmosphere results in Mrs Twentyman becoming irate and requesting a new doctor.

3 Rectal examination in abdominal pain

- Since 1901 authors have questioned the use of rectal examination in appendicitis.[10]
- It has been suggested by some authors that rectal examination in children is a specialist investigation and should only be performed in very limited situations.[11]
- One series of 323 rectal examinations in children with suspected appendicitis altered the management in just two (0.6%).
- Traditionally clinicians have been thought to examine the rectum of patients with an acute abdomen for rectal tenderness.

- In one of the largest series, 1028 patients aged between 7 and 87 with acute abdominal pain underwent rectal examination. No patients with acute appendicitis had rectal tenderness to the right in the absence of abdominal signs.[12]
- In a more recent review of 100 adults undergoing rectal examination for abdominal pain, the rectal examination did not influence the management of any patient.[13]
- Other authors have demonstrated the adverse emotional effects of rectal examination in paediatric patients.[14]

KAREN AND THE RECTAL EXAM

Clearly the evidence does not support a digital rectal examination on Karen and naturally her mother becomes upset at the suggestion. Deciding to perform such an exam would have resulted in you losing the case. Persisting in arguing your point would have ultimately led to Cahoon become irritated and taking you off call.

4 Minors and confidentiality

- Confidentiality laws will vary from region to region.
- You should be aware of the law in your area and be familar with the social support services available locally.
- From a medical perspective, your role is to support your patient as summarised in the American Academy of Pediatrics position statement,[15] which is a good medical template regardess of the region.
  - The clinican 'should not allow their personal beliefs and values to interfere with optimal patient health care'.
  - If the clinician will not counsel the patient regarding sexual matters, the patient should be referred to other experienced professionals who will.
  - The clinician should 'assess the adolescent's ability to understand the diagnosis of pregnancy and appreciate the implications of that diagnosis. The diagnosis should not be conveyed to others, including parents, until the patient's consent is obtained, except when there are concerns about suicide, homicide, or abuse'.
  - 'Adolescents should be encouraged to include their parents in a full discussion of their options.' The clinician should 'explain how parental involvement can be helpful and that parents generally are supportive'.
  - If the adolescent is reluctant to reveal the identity of the father, the paediatrician should consider the possibility of sexual abuse, sexual assault or incest.

– Usually, the adolescent has the following options available:
1. carrying her pregnancy to delivery and raising the baby
2. carrying her pregnancy to delivery and placing the baby for adoption
3. terminating her pregnancy.

KAREN AND CONFIDENTIALITY

Following the positive pregnancy test, it is your role to support Karen. Trying to impose your opinion will result in points being deducted, as will leaving Karen to solve the problem herself or asking a nurse to break the news for you. Encouraging her to involve her parents and then offering her your support while she tells her mother will earn you points. While your job as a clinician is to primarily diagnose and treat disease, you also have a responsibility to support your patient in whatever way you can. This section rewards you for doing this effectively.

5 Radiology in pregnancy

- Estimated fetal radiation doses are as follows.[16]
  Plain film of abdomen = 1.4–4.2 mGy
  Chest x-ray = <0.01 mGy
  CT abdomen = 8–49 mGy
  CT pelvis = 25–79 mGy
  Note these doses may vary per country, weight of the mother and method used.
- Digital radiography may reduce fetal radiation exposure.[17]
- Authors have suggested that gross congenital malformations will not be increased in a human pregnant population exposed to 200 mGy.[18] In a position statement over 30 years ago, the US National Council on Radiation Protection and Measurements stated: 'The risk [of abnormality] is considered to be negligible at 50 mGy or less when compared to other risks of pregnancy, and the risk of malformations is significantly increased above control levels only at doses above 150 mGy'.[19]
- Doses of radiation over 100 mGy result in a 1% increase in organ malformation and childhood cancers combined.[20]
- The UK National Radiological Protection Board has adapted an excess absolute risk (EAR) coefficient for cancer incidence under 15 years of age following low-dose irradiation *in utero* of 0.006% per mGy, compared with a risk of 0.0018% per mGy for a dose received just after birth.[21] As summarised by Lowe, this assumes that there is no threshold dose below which the risk is not increased and the risk may be greater in the first trimester than later in pregnancy.[22]

- Remember that radiation-induced effects are said to be cumulative and so it is the repeated exposure dose that is important.

KAREN AND RADIOLOGY

Bearing in mind the evidence discussed above, had you ordered radiology for Karen it is unikely that her foetus would have suffered. However, this does not escape the fact that ordering radiological investigations that are not indicated, without knowledge of whether or not your patient was pregnant, is reckless. Because of this, if you ordered such investigations you were deducted points and perhaps sent home.

6 Pregnancy tests

- A pregnancy test should be performed in all women with nausea and vomiting and of child-bearing age.[23]
- Pregnancy is the most common endocrinological cause of nausea and vomiting and must be considered in any woman of child-bearing age.[23]
- The concern with any woman with abdominal pain and a positive pregnancy test is that of an ectopic pregnancy.

KAREN AND PREGNANCY TESTS

Although young, Karen has reached menses and as such has to be considered as potentially pregnant. Given her symptoms, she required a pregnancy test. This would have speeded her diagnosis and guided your selection of medications and radiological investigations. If you failed to recognise this and ordered radiology and medications blindly, you would have lost points. Discharging her without a diagnosis would have led to her re-presenting, combined with an embarrassing situation for you professionally.

COMMUNICATION PERSPECTIVES

Nurse's perspective

- Karen is distressed and vomiting in the middle of the emergency department.
- Margaret attends a weekly meeting on the finances of the department and must answer for the department budget. The following studies have provided relevant costs.
  US 2005 study[24]:
  – 4 mg single-dose vials of ondansetron cost $26.71
  – 10 mg single-dose vials of prochlorperazine cost $9.56

– Cost per patient to be nausea and vomiting free:
  Ondansetron = $51.98
  Prochlorperazine = $13.99
UK 2002 study[25]:
– 4 mg single-dose vials of ondansetron cost £6.45
– 50 mg single-dose vials of cyclizine cost £0.54
– No clinical advantage shown, with both drugs comparable at relieving
  nausea and vomiting
• You have developed a rapport with the patient.
• Mrs Twentyman has been difficult for both nursing and medical staff to
  deal with.
• Mrs Twentyman is anxious and upon hearing that her teenage daughter is
  pregnant she may potentially become quite hostile.

SIMPSON AND THE NURSES

Eileen, who has been looking after Karen for the past 20 minutes, is
obviously anxious to help her symptoms and stop her vomiting. However,
as discussed above, it is not advisable to prescribe blindly. Margaret
becomes upset at you prescribing ondansetron. She is responsible for the
drugs budget and is often criticised by the hospital board for what is seen
as a waste of resources. As seen in the evidence above, ondansetron is
significantly more expensive than the other options, has not been shown to
be superior and as mentioned earlier is the drug with minimal experience
in pregnancy. Later in the case, you must wait 10 minutes for a nurse to
become free as a chaperone; often this is the limiting factor to using
chaperones and is an unavoidable problem in many hospitals. If you decide
to ask Eileen to tell Mrs Twentyman that her daughter is pregnant, Eileen
naturally becomes upset and complains to her superior that you are shirking
your responsibilities. She of course is right. You have built up a rapport
with Karen and telling her mother may very well turn into a difficult job as
you cannot predict how she will react, but you must be supportive of your
patient.

Karen's perspective

• Fourteen-year-old girl.
• No period for 2 months.
• Frightened.

SIMPSON AND KAREN

Karen has had no period for 2 months and when her mother is out of
earshot, tells you that she had unprotected sex with her boyfriend several

times over the past 3 months. It becomes clear that she knows that she is pregnant and has already taken a pregnancy test. She obviously did not feel comfortable telling her mother her concerns and has chosen a stranger in a relatively public place to help her. She is unsure how her mother will react and her presentation to Pilgrims emergency department is a call for help.

Mother's perspective

• Daughter is ill.
• Mother has no idea why and she is frightened.
• You are about 10 years older than her daughter.

SIMPSON AND MRS TWENTYMAN

Clearly, you have to earn Mrs Twentyman's confidence. Throughout the initial stages of the case she obviously tolerates you, just about. However, she is anxious and at any sign that you are inexperienced, she will become irate. This can be seen when you try to take a further history, or even exam her daughter. Also, to her you seem quite young and are only about 10 years older than her daughter. Furthermore, she is using displacement as a defence strategy. She is angry that Karen is unwell but cannot get angry at Karen. Instead she displaces that anger towards you. Approaching such a case, you must take these factors into consideration. Your goal is to diagnose and treat your patient and sometimes the behaviour of patients and their families can make that job harder. However, you must remain calm and sympathetic and try to earn the confidence of your patients and their families. Any other reactions only adversely affect your patient and will prevent you doing your job.

What happened to Karen?

After their initial shock, Karen's parents were very supportive, as were the parents of her boyfriend. Unfortunately Karen developed some vaginal spotting at about 13 weeks gestation and 1 week later had a spontaneous miscarriage.

DEFINITIONS

Teratogenic – an agent which causes malformations or defects in an embryo.

REFERENCE LIST

1. Gadsby R, Barnie-Adshead AM, Jagger C. A prospective study of nausea and vomiting during pregnancy. Br J Gen Pract 1993;43(371):245–248.

2. Magee LA, Mazzotta P, Koren G. Evidence-based view of safety and effectiveness of pharmacologic therapy for nausea and vomiting of pregnancy (NVP). Am J Obstet Gynecol 2002;186(5 Suppl Understanding):S256–S261.

3. Seto A, Einarson T, Koren G. Pregnancy outcome following first trimester exposure to antihistamines: meta-analysis. Am J Perinatol 1997;14(3):119–124.

4. Tucker ML, Jackson MR, Scales MD, Spurling NW, Tweats DJ, Capel-Edwards K. Ondansetron: pre-clinical safety evaluation. Eur J Cancer Clin Oncol 1989;25(Suppl 1):S79–S93.

5. Sullivan CA, Johnson CA, Roach H, Martin RW, Stewart DK, Morrison JC. A pilot study of intravenous ondansetron for hyperemesis gravidarum. Am J Obstet Gynecol 1996;174(5):1565–1568.

6. Jewell D, Young G. Interventions for nausea and vomiting in early pregnancy. Cochrane Database Syst Rev 2003;4:CD000145.

7. American Academy of Pediatrics Committee on Practice and Ambulatory Medicine. The use of chaperones during the physical examination of the pediatric patient. Pediatrics 1996;98(6 pt 1):1202.

8. Ehrenthal DB, Farber NJ, Collier VU, Aboff BM. Chaperone use by residents during pelvic, breast, testicular, and rectal exams. J Gen Intern Med 2000;15(8):573–576.

9. Penn MA, Bourguet CC. Patients' attitudes regarding chaperones during physical examinations. J Fam Pract 1992;35(6):639–643.

10. Osler W. The Principles and Practices of Medicine Designed for the Use of Practitioners and Students of Medicine. New York: Appleton, 1901.

11. Jesudason EC, Walker J. Rectal examination in paediatric surgical practice. Br J Surg 1999;86(3):376–378.

12. Dixon JM, Elton RA, Rainey JB, Macleod DA. Rectal examination in patients with pain in the right lower quadrant of the abdomen. BMJ 1991;302(6773):386–388.

13. Manimaran RG. Significance of routine digital rectal examination in adults presenting with abdominal pain. Ann R Coll Surg Engl 2004;86:292–295.

14. Rockney RM, McQuade WH, Days AL. The plain abdominal roentgenogram in the management of encopresis. Arch Pediatr Adolesc Med 1995;149(6):623–627.

15. American Academy of Pediatrics Committee on Adolescence. Counseling the adolescent about pregnancy options. Pediatrics 1998;101(5):938–940.

16. Valentin J. Pregnancy and Medical Radiation. Ann ICRP 2000;30:1–43.

17. Claussen C, Kohler D, Christ F, Golde G, Lochner B. Pelvimetry by digital radiography and its dosimetry. J Perinat Med 1985;13(6):287–292.

18. Brent RL. Utilization of developmental basic science principles in the evaluation of reproductive risks from pre- and postconception environmental radiation exposures. Teratology 1999;59(4):182–204.

19. National Council on Radiation Protection and Measurements. Medical Radiation Exposure of Pregnant and Potentially Pregnant Women. NCRP Report No. 54. Bethesda, MD: National Council on Radiation Protection and Measurements, 1977.

20. McCollough CH, Schueler BA, Atwell TD, et al. Radiation exposure and pregnancy: when should we be concerned? Radiographics 2007;27(4):909–917.

21. Sharp C, Shrimpton JA, Bury RF. Diagnostic Medical Exposures: Advice on Exposure to Ionizing Radiation During Pregnancy. Chilton, Oxon: National Radiological Protection Board, 1998.

22. Lowe SA. Diagnostic radiography in pregnancy: risks and reality. Aust NZ J Obstet Gynaecol 2004;44(3):191–196.

23. Scorza K, Williams A, Phillips JD, Shaw J. Evaluation of nausea and vomiting. Am Fam Physician 2007;76(1):76–84.

24. Chang P, Okamoto M, Chen J, Frame D. Cost-effectiveness analysis of ondansetron and prochlorperazine for the prevention of postoperative nausea and vomiting. J Manag Care Pharm 2005;11(4):317–321.

25. Grimsehl K, Whiteside JB, Mackenzie N. Comparison of cyclizine and ondansetron for the prevention of postoperative nausea and vomiting in laparoscopic day-case gynaecological surgery. Anaesthesia 2002;57(1):61–65.

Case perspectives: Sharyn Romanowska

THERAPEUTIC PERSPECTIVES

1 Analgesia

Stabilising the patient and relieving pain must be the doctor's priority. This concept has been recognised legally with the James and Bergman cases,* where juries awarded $16.5 million to patients where medical staff did not adequately treat their pain.

We should all be familiar with the World Health Organisation's analgesic ladder.[1]

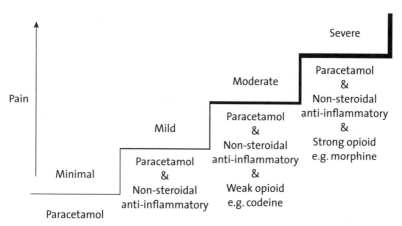

WHO analgesic ladder.

APPROACHES TO ANALGESIA

PARACETAMOL/ACETAMINOPHEN
Adverse effects are rare in safe doses; however, larger doses can result in side-effects.

Side-effects: paracetamol/acetaminophen

• Nausea and vomiting
• Diarrhoea
• Seizures

*please refer to the Definitions at the end of this Case perspective.

- Renal failure
- Liver failure
- Abdominal pain

NON-STEROIDAL ANTI-INFLAMMATORIES (NSAIDS)

Excellent analgesic properties, but often considered 'dirty' drugs because of the safety profile of some of the stronger NSAIDs such as diclofenac.

Side-effects: NSAIDs

- Nausea and vomiting
- Diarrhoea
- Upper GI irritation
- Bleeding tendency
- Rash
- Constipation
- Renal failure
- Respiratory distress (asthmatics)
- Reye's syndrome (aspirin)*

MORPHINE/OPIOIDS

Intravenous morphine is the gold standard in analgesia. Its effects are quick but it is short acting.

Side-effects: opioids

- Respiratory depression
- Nausea and vomiting
- Itch
- Addiction
- Sedation
- Cough suppression
- Urinary retention

NUMBERS NEEDED TO TREAT

Although it has its limitations, the concept of 'numbers needed to treat'* (number of patients needed to be given the drug to provide a 50% reduction in pain) is useful when deciding upon your analgesic strategy (Table 1).

Table 1 The 2007 Oxford league table of analgesic efficacy (modified)[2]

Analgesic (mg)*	NNT**
Diclofenac 100	1.8
Paracetamol/acetaminophen 1000 + codeine 60	2.2
Aspirin 1200	2.4
Ibuprofen 400	2.5
Diclofenac 25	2.6
Ibuprofen 200	2.7
Pethidine 100 (intramuscular)	2.9
Tramadol 150	2.9
Morphine 10 (intramuscular)	2.9
Ibuprofen 100	3.7
Paracetamol/acetaminophen 1000	3.8
Ibuprofen 50	4.7
Tramadol 100	4.8
Paracetamol/acetaminophen 300 + codeine 30	5.7
Tramadol 50	8.3
Codeine 60	16.7

*Administered orally unless otherwise stated.
**Numbers needed to treat.

SHARYN AND ANALGESIA

Sharyn was exhibiting signs of peritonism secondary to a duodenal perforation caused by NSAIDs. Although an effective adjunct, paracetamol/acetaminophen would not be sufficient to control her pain. If you choose this alone, you would have lost points as it was insufficient.

Apart from the obvious cause and effect link with NSAIDs, Sharyn's blood tests demonstrate impaired renal function, most likely secondary to shock. The addition of NSAIDs may put her kidneys under further strain, and would also result in you being penalised.

Intravenous morphine, while simultaneously rehydrating her, would help control her symptoms. Although traditionally there have been concerns that morphine causes hypotension, this effect appears to be overstated, and its use while also addressing Sharyn's dehydration would be a sensible strategy. As morphine also causes nausea and vomiting, a morphine and antiemetic combination would be advised.

2 Fluid resuscitation

- Crystalloid (isotonic), colloid and hypertonic fluids* have all been used in fluid resuscitation.
- Currently crystalloid isotonic fluids are the resuscitation fluid of choice.
- Sharyn has been vomiting for 5 hours and is profoundly dehydrated. The attending doctor must remember to supplement her potassium and monitor her electrolytes.
- Perforated peptic ulcer disease carries a mortality of approximately 10% and even higher in the elderly population.[3] The factors that influence this are:
  - greater than 12 hours of symptoms
  - shock
  - patients older than 75 years
  - co-morbidities.

  Sharyn has two out of these four factors. Adequate fluid resuscitation will be crucial for her survival. This should be done prior to surgical intervention.
- Sharyn also has concomitant cardiac disease. This will make her fluid resuscitation more complex, as you will have to monitor her carefully for fluid overload. Ideally this should be done in the ICU with central venous pressure and urine output monitoring.

SHARYN AND FLUID RESUSCITATION

In this case if you attempted to bring Sharyn to theatre without adequately resuscitating her, you lost points. Sharyn would have arrested intraoperatively if no resuscitation had taken place, or would have developed renal failure postoperatively, requiring dialyisis.

3 Imaging

- A plain film of abdomen is a diagnostic test with a very poor yield in most clinical situations. It has been shown to alter the diagnosis in 7% of abdominal pains, and actually alter management in just 4%.[4]
- An erect chest x-ray has a sensitivity of 78% for demonstrating a perforation. If the patient is unable to sit up for the required time, a left lateral decubitus film* can also help. Studies have suggested that ultrasound has a sensitivity* of 92% for free air, but currently this is not in standard use.[5]
- CT scanning has a sensitivity approaching 100% for free air. However, unlike a plain film or ultrasound, CT requires that the patient must

physically leave the relative safety of the resuscitation room to travel to the CT machine. This is a potentially dangerous period and the patient must be stable enough to be moved. For this reason, the CT machine has earned the unfortunate nickname of 'the doughnut of death'.

SHARYN AND IMAGING

If you requested a plain film of abdomen for Sharyn, you would have been penalised. In this case it is vital to prioritise your investigations to get the important information both quickly and safely. Similarly, if you sent Sharyn for a CT scan without first stabilising her, she went on to arrest within the CT machine and die later in the ICU. Like everything else in clinical practice, choosing your investigations is not simply a matter of picking the textbook 'best test'; you must take into account the picture in front of you.

4 Conservative versus operative management

- In approximately 50% of patients the perforation has sealed by the time of presentation.[6] CT will not tell you this as it will only show free air. Contrast radiology with water-soluble contrast* (not barium) is used to answer this question.

- In recent years the conservative management of perforated ulcers has become more established, particularly if you consider that up to 50 % of perforations will have sealed by presentation.[7] However, Sharyn has generalised peritonitis with a large pneumoperitoneum. In this picture it is very hard to argue against surgery following adequate resuscitation.

- In other cases where the patient is not peritonitic and you decide on a trial of conservative treatment, you would:
  - resuscitate
  - administer analgesia
  - decompress the stomach with a nasogastric tube
  - administer broad-spectrum antibiotics
  - monitor closely.

SHARYN AND CONSERVATIVE TREATMENT

If you decided on a trial of conservative treatment with Sharyn, she would have deteriorated. At this stage if you still persisted with a conservative approach, she would have died.

5 Laparoscopic versus open

- Outcome studies vary but generally laparoscopy requires less analgesia postoperatively.[8]

- Laparoscopy is difficult and potentially dangerous in patients who have had previous abdominal surgery. The first difficulty is getting your first port into the peritoneum safely. Even if this is achieved, it is often impossible to get a good visualisation if there are widespread adhesions.

SHARYN AND LAPAROSCOPY

In Sharyn's case a laparoscopic approach was doomed to failure given her extensive previous surgery. Trying to persist with laparoscopy in such a hostile peritoneum would add a considerable amount of time to surgery in quite a sick patient.

COMMUNICATION PERSPECTIVES

Nurse's perspective

- Margaret is the head nurse.
- She has four nurses off sick and management has given her just two replacement nurses. Neither has ever worked in the emergency department. You would not have been aware of this.
- A patient stalled in the resuscitation room ties up at least one of her experienced staff for potentially hours. Outside the patients are mounting up.
- In her experience, patients with perforated ulcers go to theatre; therefore she puts incredible pressure on you to move the patient quickly, feeling that this is in the best interest of the patient and the department. She becomes frustrated when you delay moving the patient.

SIMPSON AND MARGARET

The key to Sharyn's survival is resuscitation. You're trained to specifically look after this type of patient and must be aware of this. Part of working with your colleagues is communicating effectively and appreciating your colleagues' perspective. You were penalised if you became distracted by Margaret's comments as arguing distracts everybody from the most important job, that of looking after Sharyn.

Husband's perspective

- Sharyn's husband, Stefan, had been through a considerable amount with his wife of 34 years. She has had multiple admissions with her COPD and inflammatory bowel disease. She has also had a small bowel and large bowel resection, along with a cholecystectomy.

- He was terrified that she would require further surgery.
- He tries to rationalise* her symptoms by insisting that they were caused by the chicken they bought from the local butchers.
- Clearly Sharyn's symptoms are not due to food poisioning.

SIMPSON AND STEFAN

Patients and their relatives often try to rationalise and explain symptoms in a way that makes sense to them. Medicine is a completely foreign and terryifying subject to most patients. While it is imperative to listen carefully, as the diagnosis is often in what you are told, it is important to remain objective, weighing up what you see in front of you with what the patient, relatives and your investigations tell you.

What happened to Sharyn?

Sharyn was resuscitated and following this, she was brought to theatre for a laparotomy. Upon opening her peritoneum, we found dense adhesions. The adhesions were taken down and we found a perforation in her duodenum. This was oversewn using a patch from her omentum. Sharyn was returned to the ICU postoperatively and was kept ventilated overnight. The following day her ECG demonstrated new T-wave inversion indicative of ischaemia. She developed heart failure complicated by renal failure and unfortunately died 3 days later.

DEFINITIONS

James and Bergman cases – in 1991 a North Carolina jury awarded $15 million to the family of Henry James who was a nursing home patient with metastatic prostate cancer. The jury concluded that a nurse's refusal to administer opioid analgesia represented a gross departure from medical care. In 1998 a jury in California concluded that upon discharge from hospital, patient William Berman had inadequate pain relief. On the day of discharge, a pain score of 10 was recorded in his chart, with his score fluctuating between 7 and 10 throughout his stay. Declining further tests, he returned home and died 1 week later. His family were awarded $1.5 million under the elder abuse statute.

Reyes syndrome is a rare disorder mainly affecting those under the age of 15. It is characterized by brain and liver damage following a viral infection such as chickenpox or influenza. It may also be linked to taking aspirin to treat a viral infection.

Numbers needed to treat – the number of patients who need to be treated to prevent one bad outcome.

Hypertonic fluids – the most commonly studied fluid of this type is 7.5% sodium chloride. Although licensed by the American military, it is still experimental in civilian use.

Left lateral decubitus film – a plain film with the patient lying on their left side. Free air should rise and if present will be seen at the top of the radiograph. Left is chosen in order to avoid confusion with the gastric bubble.

Sensitivity – the proportion of people with disease (free air in this case) who have a positive test. Compare this with **specificity** – the proportion of people without the disease (no free air) who have a negative test.

Water-soluble contrast agent – agents swallowed or injected which allow visualisation of a system or organ through radiographic scanning. Traditionally contrast materials have been iodine-based agents but these are irritant, especially to the peritoneum. Thus where a perforation is suspected, the less irritant water-soluble agents are used.

Rationalisation – the cognitive process of making something seem consistent with or based on reason.

REFERENCE LIST

1. World Health Organisation's analgesic ladder. WHO website. Available at http://www.who.int/cancer/palliative/painladder/en/. Accessed April 12, 2010.

2. Oxford League Table of Analgesics in Acute Pain. Bandolier Web site. Available at: http://www.medicine.ox.ac.uk/bandolier/booth/painpag/acutrev/analgesics/lftab.html. Accessed April 12, 2010.

3. Svances C. Trends in perforated peptic ulcer: incidence, etiology, treatment and prognosis. *Worls J Surg* 2000;24:277–83.

4. Stower MJ, Amar SS, Mikulin T, Kean DM, Hardcastle JD. Evaluation of the plain abdominal X-ray in the acute abdomen. J R Soc Med 1985;78(8):630–633.

5. Chen S-C, Yen Z-S, Wang H-P, Lin F-Y, Hsu C-Y, Chen W-J. Ultrasonography is superior to plain radiology in the diagnosis of pneumoperitoneum. Br J Surg 2002;89:351–4.

6. Crofts TJ, Park KG, Steele RJ, Chung SS, Li AK. A randomized trial of nonoperative treatment for perforated peptic ulcer. N Engl J Med 1989;320(15):970–973.

7. Donovan AJ, Berne TV, Donovan JA. Perforated duodenal ulcer: an alternative therapeutic plan. Arch Surg 1998;133:166–71.

8. Siu WT, Leong HT, Law BK et al. Laparoscopic repair for perforated peptic ulcer: a randomised controlled trial. Ann Surg 2002;235:313–19.

Case perspectives: Jill Baruani

THERAPEUTIC PERSPECTIVES

1 Pressure to stop bleeding

The first steps in managing this patient's bleeding are pressure and elevation. In general, you should approach any bleeding outside theatre in a stepwise fashion (see below), always starting with compression.[1]

Apply direct pressure & elevate limb

Pack wound

Windlass technique
A dressing is applied directly to the wound and held in place by a broad bandage with a knot over the wound. A pen or other similar object is then placed under the knot and rotated until tight. It is then secured providing significant direct pressure

↓

Indirect pressure

↓

Use of a tourniquet

Note: Topical haemostatic agents can be added at any stage

Stepwise approach to managing bleeding.

Suturing blindly into a wound is often dangerous, especially as bleeding tends to obscure your vision. This risks injury to surrounding structures, depending on the site and circumstances of bleeding. In this case, the bleeding from a stab avulsion site was likely to be quite superficial and you were not docked points for placing a stitch. However, maximum marks were awarded for using pressure to arrest the bleeding.

2 Application of a tourniquet

Tourniquets have been demonstrasted to have a role in massive haemorrhage from extremities in a military setting.[2] It has been speculated that their use in the Vietnam war may have prevented 7% of combat deaths.[3] However, while tourniquets may have a role in controlling catastrophic limb bleeding, they are not without complications and their uses in civilian life are limited to a very small number of prehospital settings.

- Extreme life-threatening limb haemorrhage or limb amputation/mangled limb with multiple bleeding points, to allow immediate management of airway and breathing problems.
- Life-threatening limb haemorrhage not controlled by simple methods.
- Point of significant haemorrhage from limb is not peripherally accessible due to entrapment.
- Major incident or multiple casualties with extremity haemorrhage and lack of resources to maintain simple methods of haemorrhage control.
- Benefits of preventing death from hypovolaemic shock by cessation of ongoing external haemorrhage are greater than the risk of limb damage or loss from ischaemia caused by tourniquet use.[1]

  There are several problems associated with tourniquet use.

- The occlusion of arterial blood flow to a limb results in ischaemia with nerve injury and possibly compartment syndrome at 2 hours and permanent muscle loss at 6 hours.[4]
- Pain.
- Reperfusion injury – the limb accumulates proinflammatory agents during ischaemia. These are then released systemically following reperfusion. The resulting inflammatory response causes inflammation and oxidative damage.

In short, although tourniquets may have a role in the military and in a few select civilian circumstances, they would not be indicated in this case. The patient's bleeding could have easily been arrested by simple compression helped by elevation, with minimal adverse affects. If you chose to use a tourniquet, you would have lost points.

COMMUNICATION PERSPECTIVES

Nurse's perspective

- Caroline is the ward nurse looking after Jill's postoperative care.
- She has worked on the wards for about 5 years.
- Like Cahoon, this is her first night working with you.

- She is familiar with what doctors have done in the past to manage similar problems.
- She has never seen a tourniquet being used in this situation before.

SIMPSON AND CAROLINE

Caroline's priority, as yours, is the patient. She has never seen a tourniquet being used on a ward before, particularly in the setting of such a controllable bleed. If you decided to apply a tourniquet, she becomes concerned, especially when the patient becomes distressed with pain. Quite rightly, she seeks the advice of your senior colleague, and is ultimately proved correct. Like Cahoon, and every colleague, she must learn to trust you.

Intern's perspective

- This is Mia's first job and like you, she is uncertain and anxious.
- She is right to expect senior help.
- You have no experience of her clinical skills.

SIMPSON AND MIA CHANG

You need to recognise that Mia is very new to the job and as such needs your help. This protects Mia and, most importantly, protects your patient. Until you are comfortable that she can deal with problems on her own, she needs to be encouraged to call you. If you ignored her request for help, you were docked points. It is likely that in a few weeks she would deal effectively with this problem herself, but for now she needs supervision and support.

Cahoon's perspective

- Cahoon is the senior trainee on call tonight.
- He is responsible for the safety of the surgical patients on the wards, in theatre and in A&E.
- It is his first night on call with you, and he has no opinion of your clinical skills yet.

SIMPSON AND CAHOON

Cahoon must first see that he can trust you to be safe. If you did not respond to the intern's call, you were deducted points, as clearly there was a potential problem on the ward and you failed to recognise it. Even if you were not confident enough to solve the problem yourself, you should have recognised the potential danger and let him know you were out of your depth. This was achieved by applying pressure and looking for senior help.

Obviously, solving the problem itself gained you maximum marks. The more your senior colleagues can trust you, the more you can achieve in a job. This starts first with demonstrating that you are safe.

What happened to Jill?

Jill had no further bleeding and recovered well. She was very happy with the result and returned 8 weeks later for surgery for the varicose veins on her other leg.

REFERENCE LIST

1. Lee C, Porter KM, Hodgetts TJ. Tourniquet use in the civilian prehospital setting. Emerg Med J 2007;24(8):584–587.

2. Kragh JF Jr, Walters TJ, Baer DG, et al. Survival with emergency tourniquet use to stop bleeding in major limb trauma. Ann Surg 2009;249(1):1–7.

3. Bellamy RF. Combat trauma overview. In: Zajtchuk R, Grande CM, (eds) *Textbook of Military Medicine Part IV: Surgical Combat Casualty Care*. Falls Church, VA: Office of the Surgeon General, US Army, 2005.

4. Wakai A, Winter DC, Street JT, Redmond PH. Pneumatic tourniquets in extremity surgery. J Am Acad Orthop Surg 2001;9(5):345–351.

Case perspectives: Trent Goeken

THERAPEUTIC PERSPECTIVES

1 Antibiotics

- Antibiotic penetration is usually very poor into an abscess cavity as the cavity lacks a blood supply.
- The evidence has established that there is no difference in outcomes between those immunocompetent patients given antibiotics and those not,[1,2] after the abscess had been drained.

TRENT AND ANTIBIOTICS

Trent had a well-established abscess from a sebaceous cyst. The antibiotics prescribed by his family doctor had not helped. Therefore persisting with this form of treatment resulted in points being deducted.

Similarly, the evidence does not support the use of antibiotics after the abscess has been drained. If you prescribed these, you were also docked points.

2 Local anaesthetic

- Local anesthetic works poorly in areas of low pH, such as found within an abscess cavity.
- Overall, the evidence in this area is poor.
- Some reseachers advocate using local anaesthetic in the skin around the abscess[3]; another alternative is a regional block.*
- Patients generally feel the most discomfort during the breakdown of loculations* rather than the incision itself.[4]

TRENT AND ANAESTHETIC

Injecting the local anaesthetic directly into the abscess cavity was not effective and you would have been deducted points. Attempting to infiltrate the area around the site would have gained you points. While a GA offers complete comfort, there are other complications associated with general anaesthesia as well as logistical considerations.

3 Culturing

Sending the pus for culture and sensitivity does not affect the management or clinical outcome in immunocompetent patients.[5,6]

*please refer to the Definitions at the end of this Case perspective.

TRENT AND CULTURING

If you requested a culture and sensitivity on the pus, you were deducted points. The evidence does not support routine culturing, it adds to the workload of the microbiology department and is a waste of funds.

4 Follow-up

The abscess may destroy the underlying sebaceous cyst* but the cyst can also remain and potentially be a source of another abscess.

TRENT AND FOLLOW-UP

If you did not follow up Trent, he re-presented 2 months later with another abscess and you were deducted points. It is worth examining the area to ensure that the source of the abscess (the cyst) has been destroyed.

COMMUNICATION PERSPECTIVES

Trent's perspective

• Trent has had a sebaceous cyst for many years without seeking attention.
• This is the first time it has given him a problem.

SIMPSON AND TRENT

Patients often want to be educated about their conditions, as well as encouraged to learn more. In this instance, Trent was happy to trust your advice regarding anaesthetic, antibiotics and follow-up. Making sure your advice is correct and evidence based should be your priority.

What happened to Trent?

Trent returned to outpatients 6 weeks later and a small residual cyst was noted. He had the non-infected cyst excised under local anaesthetic the following day and experienced no further problems.

DEFINITIONS

Loculations – in this setting, loculations are pockets of pus divided into small cavities or compartments within the cavity.

Regional block – a method of anaesthesia used to anaesthetise parts, or regions, of the body without the patient going to sleep.

Sebaceous cyst – a common cyst of skin formed by distension of a sebaceous gland due to obstruction of its excretory duct.

REFERENCE LIST

1. Meislin HW, Lerner SA, Graves MH, et al. Cutaneous abscesses. Anaerobic and aerobic bacteriology and outpatient management. Ann Intern Med 1977;87(2):145–149.

2. Llera JL, Levy RC. Treatment of cutaneous abscess: a double-blind clinical study. Ann Emerg Med 1985;14(1):15–19.

3. Derksen DJ. Pfenninger and Fowler's Procedures for Primary Care, 2nd edn. St Louis, MO: Mosby, 2009.

4. Halvorson GD, Halvorson JE, Iserson KV. Abscess incision and drainage in the emergency department. Part I. J Emerg Med 1985;3(3):227–232.

5. Garcea G, Lloyd T, Jacobs M, Cope A, Swann A, Berry D. Role of microbiological investigations in the management of non-perineal cutaneous abscesses. Postgrad Med J 2003;79(935):519–521.

6. Khan MN, Vidya R, Lee RE. The limited role of microbiological culture and sensitivity in the management of superficial soft tissue abscesses. Sci World J 2006;6:1118–1123.

Case perspectives: David Cummins

THERAPEUTIC PERSPECTIVES

1 ABCs

- The ATLS©* protocol teaches that death due to trauma occurs in one of three time periods.

  1. Seconds to minutes after injury – often these patients are impossible to save. It includes injuries such as lacerations to major vessels, brainstem, heart, etc.

  2. Minutes to hours after injury – this is the period which is the primary focus of the ATLS© guidelines. It includes lacerations to liver or spleen, pneumothorax,* pelvic fractures.

  3. Days to weeks after injury – this period is often the realm of the intensive care setting. It includes patients with sepsis and multi-organ failure. This period is dependent on the results of the second time period.

- The airway is assessed first in your primary survey. If the patient is able to communicate verbally, it is unlikely that there is an immediate threat to airway patency. However, reassessment is imperative. Furthermore, speaking to the patient allows you to assess his/her GCS* as well as getting an idea of the mechanism of injury. During the initial assessment of the airway, it is essential to ensure that the patients' cervical collar has been stabilised and secured.

- Next, you must ensure that the patient is oxygenating themselves adequately by inspecting, palpating, percussing and listening. Adjuncts such as pulse oximetery* also help but should be interpreted with care in the shocked patient.

- The next part of your primary survey is to assess your patient's circulation. If the patient has been verbalising then they are perfusing their brain. Watch for the patient's colour (pink is generally perfused, grey or white is a sign of shock), and of course assess their pulse, its rate and quality. Care must be taken with an apparently normal BP reading, as often BP is preserved until late in shock (Table 2). Also, some medications (for example, beta-blockers) can prevent a compensatory tachycardia and previde erroneous reassurance.

*please refer to the Definitions at the end of this Case perspective.

Table 2 Classification of shock (ATLS©)

	Class 1	Class 2	Class 3	Class 4
Blood loss (ml)	Up to 750	750–1500	1500–2000	>2000
Blood loss (%)	Up to 15%	15–30%	30–40%	>40%
Pulse rate	<100	>100	>120	>140
Blood pressure	Normal	Normal	Decreased	Decreased
Pulse pressure*	Normal (or increased)	Decreased	Decreased	Decreased
Respiratory rate	14–20	20–30	30–40	>35
Urine output (ml/hour)	>30	20–30	5–15	Negligible
Mental status	Slightly anxious	Mildly anxious	Anxious or confused	Confused and lethargic

- How patients respond to fluid resuscitation is a guide to their ultimate management (Table 3).

Table 3 The patient's response to fluids as a guide to management (modified from ATLS©)

	Rapid responder	Transient responder	No response
Vital signs	Return to normal	Transient response but quick rise in pulse or fall in BP	Remain abnormal
Estimated blood loss	Minimal (10–20%)	Moderate and ongoing (20–40%)	Severe (>40%)
Need for blood	Low	High	Immediate
Blood preparation	Type and crossmatch	Type specific	Emergency blood needed
Need for operative intervention	Possibly	Likely	Highly likely
Early presence of surgeon	Yes	Yes	Yes

DAVID AND ABCS

Your first challenge was to manage David's primary assessment. Taking each element of this in the right order earned you a point. If you deviated significantly, for example such as inserting a urinary catheter, before adequately assessing the airway and breathing, you were deducted points.

His pulse was initally 106 with a BP of 130/84. In this setting, he was at worst a class 2 shock. However, ultimately he responded to fluids and was a 'rapid responder'.

2 Pneumothorax and theatre

- An unrecognised pneumothorax can be converted into a life-threatening tension pneumothorax during general anaesthesia.
- This can be a result of positive pressure ventilation and the use of nitrous oxide.*
- If there is air in the pleural space, nitrous oxide in the blood can diffuse rapidly into the area due to the differential solubility between nitrous oxide and nitrogen. This can cause a doubling in the pneumothorax volume within 10 minutes.[1]
- Whatever the mechanism, as the air in the pleural space increases, it causes progressive vena caval obstruction, decreased blood return to the heart, tachycardia, hypotension and eventually death.

DAVID AND PNEUMOTHORAX

Failing to assess David's ABCs led to a deduction of points as it represents a serious error in trauma management. Not following ATLS protocol resulted in your patient having a pneumothorax which is eventually spotted by Nicola Pablo, your anaesthetist, who complains to Cahoon that you're not safe, failing to diagnose David's pneumothorax, with potentially life-threatening consequences.

3 Wide-bore cannula

- Attempted cannulation should begin with peripheral access as per ATLS© protocols, with two wide-bore cannulae (14 gauge).
- Peripheral cannulation is generally quicker than central access and is thus preferred initially where possible.
- Hagen–Poiseuille's law governs flow through a tubular structure. Flow rate is proportional to the fourth power of the radius of the tube, and inversely proportional to its length. In summary, short and wide is good, long and narrow bad.
- Triple-lumen central lines often have two 18 G and one 16 G lumen, while the single-lumen central line is generally a 14 G.
- Central lines are longer than peripheral lines (~10 cm vs ~2 cm).
- The lower the gauge, the wider the cannula lumen. Hence a 14 G has a wider lumen than a 16 G or 18 G.
- This gauge system is an old way of measuring lumen size based on the lumen being '14th of an inch in diameter', hence 14 G.

- For all these reasons, it is clear that two 14 G peripheral lines (shorter and wider) are preferable to a triple- or even single-lumen central line, when resuscitation is required (Table 4).

Table 4 Peripheral versus central access for resuscitation

Peripheral access	Central access
Shorter	Longer
Wider	Narrower
Quicker to insert	Slower to insert
Two separate lines	One single- or triple-lumen line

Central lines do have advantages over peripheral lines in other situations (Table 5).

Table 5 Advantages and disadvantages of central lines

Advantages	Disadvantages
Durable	Thrombosis
Infuse irritants (chemo, TPN, inotropes)	Inferior flow rates to wide-bore peripheral lines in resuscitation
Invasive monitoring (CVP)	Insertion complications
Allows easy blood withdrawal	Serious infection/sepsis risk
	More skill required to insert

When it comes to choosing your site for a central line, there is little evidence to favour subclavian over jugular lines. However, there is clear evidence to favour subclavian lines over femoral lines, with subclavian lines having fewer[2] infectious and mechanical/insertion complications, and less thrombosis.

DAVID AND WIDE-BORE CANNULA

In David's case, it is clear that you should have attempted peripheral access first. If you decided to opt for central access first, your attempts would have been interrupted by a senior emergency department colleague, who took over the care of the patient. For this, you would have been deducted points.

4 Imaging

- Ultrasound is quick, non-invasive and can be performed at the bedside. However, it is user dependent and very poor for hollow viscus injury.
- Ultrasound has a sensitivity of 88%, a specificity of 99% and an accuracy of 97% for detecting intra-abdominal injuries in blunt trauma.[3] However, it

can miss small amounts of intraperitoneal fluid. Overall, it is not as reliable in penetrating injuries.[4]

- CT is organ specific and does provide imaging of retroperitoneal structures. However, it does require that the patient is stable and ideally will require contrast medium.
- Even with modern multidetector machines, CT is still weak at identifying diaphram, mesenteric and hollow viscus injuries.[5]

DAVID AND IMAGING

If you ordered a CT without resuscitating your patient properly, he would have arrested in radiology and required emergency laparotomy. This is an incredibly serious mistake and for this you would have been dismissed from duties by Cahoon. Choosing an ultrasound would have given you a normal result as is sometimes the case in user-dependent investigations. However, you would not have been deducted points as it is a reasonable test in a potentially unstable patient and your descision to intervene still remained clinical. A CT would have shown you a small amount of free air and fluid. This resulted from the breach in peritoneum from the stab wound. However, again, like the ultrasound, your descision to intervene still remains clinical.

5 Conservative versus operative management

- It has been observed that a negative laparotomy will occur in 23–57% cases of penetrating abdominal trauma.[6,7]
- The rate of complications with a negative laparotomy has been estimated to be up to 27%.[8]
- Due to the high morbidity, many centres practise a mandatory laparotomy for abdominal gunshot wounds.[9]
- Although recent studies have challenged some of the traditional indications for laparotomy in the setting of penetrating trauma outside of gunshot wounds, as a rule of thumb the following are considered indications for laparotomy[10]: peritonitis, haemodynamic instability.
- The following have been considered relative indications for laparotomy[10]: isolated evisceration* retained foreign bodies.

DAVID AND CONSERVATIVE TREATMENT

If you decided on a trial of conservative treatment with David, he would have deteriorated, exhibiting a tachycardia. Attributing this tachycardia to pain alone and failing to reassess resulted in David becoming shocked. While there is certainly a role for conservative treatment in penetrating abdominal injury, failing to recognise that this patient was developing shock would have resulted in points deduction.

6 Laparoscopic versus open

- Laparoscopy is especially suited to scenarios where there may be peritoneal penetration (as in David's case) or those injuries that CT may miss such as diaphragmatic injuries or mesenteric haematomas.[11]
- Laparoscopy is not useful for assessing retroperitoneal organs or structures.

DAVID AND LAPAROSCOPY

If you chose to perform a laparoscopy you received maximum marks. If instead you opted for a laparotomy, you were certainly not wrong and were awarded points. However, Cahoon would have suggested first starting with a laparoscopy.

COMMUNICATION PERSPECTIVES

Nurse's perspective

Izzy is involved in three ways.

1. She reminds you to assess the patient properly before catheterising.
2. She reports her concerns to Margaret when you miss the pneumothorax.
3. She takes her break and is replaced by another nurse.

SIMPSON AND IZZY

You should use whatever experience is available in the department. Izzy was right to report her concerns to senior staff when you made the fundamental error of not assessing David's ABCs. Although you are primarily responsible for David regardless of where he is, nursing staff run an effective shift system which generally works well to ensure breaks can be rotated. However, this case emphasises how this system can fail, especially in a busy unit, regardless of how prestigious it might be. Human error and staff looking after too many patients can result in important signs being overlooked.

What happened to David?

David reported that he had been robbed and stabbed with a screwdriver. However, his abdominal wound was tangential and quite clean. As it transpired, he was involved in selling heroin and had been stabbed by a rival drug dealer. Although he recovered from the stab wound, being discharged on day 4 post op, he was fatally shot 3 months later.

DEFINITIONS

ATLS – Advanced Trauma and Life Support. ATLS is the protocol and standard of care for the initial assessment and treatment of trauma. It is used in over 40 different countries.

Pneumothorax – abnormal presence of air in the pleural cavity resulting in the collapse of the lung.

GCS – Glasgow Coma Scale. Standardised rating system used to evaluate the degree of consciousness impairment based on eye opening, motor response and verbal response.

Pulse oximetry – a non-invasive and painless way to measure the oxygen saturation of arterial blood.

Pulse pressure – the difference between systolic and diastolic blood pressures.

Nitrous oxide – (N_2O) a non-flammable gas used in surgery and dentistry for its anaesthetic effects.

Evisceration – the exteriorising of some or all of the vital organs, usually from the abdomen.

REFERENCE LIST

1. Eger EI, Saidman LJ. Hazards of nitrous oxide anesthesia in bowel obstruction and pneumothorax. Anesthesiology 1965;26:61–66.

2. Hamilton HC, Foxcroft D. Central venous access sites for the prevention of venous thrombosis, stenosis and infection in patients requiring long-term intravenous therapy. Cochrane Database Syst Rev 2007;3:CD004084.

3. McKenney MG, Martin L, Lentz K, et al. 1,000 consecutive ultrasounds for blunt abdominal trauma. J Trauma 1996;40(4):607–610.

4. Udobi KF, Rodriguez A, Chiu WC, Scalea TM. Role of ultrasonography in penetrating abdominal trauma: a prospective clinical study. J Trauma 2001;50(3):475–479.

5. Ekeh AP, Saxe J, Walusimbi M, et al. Diagnosis of blunt intestinal and mesenteric injury in the era of multidetector CT technology – are results better? J Trauma 2008;65(2):354–359.

6. Ross SE, Dragon GM, O'Malley KF, Rehm CG. Morbidity of negative coeliotomy in trauma. Injury 1995;26(6):393–394.

7. Leppaniemi A, Salo J, Haapiainen R. Complications of negative laparotomy for truncal stab wounds. J Trauma 1995;38(1):54–58.

8. Weigelt JA, Kingman RG. Complications of negative laparotomy for trauma. Am J Surg 1988;156(6):544–547.

9. Muckart DJ, Abdool-Carrim AT, King B. Selective conservative management of abdominal gunshot wounds: a prospective study. Br J Surg 1990;77(6):652–655.

10. Clarke SC, Stearns AT, Payne C, McKay AJ. The impact of published recommendations on the management of penetrating abdominal injury. Br J Surg 2008;95(4):515–521.

11. Fabian TC, Croce MA, Stewart RM, Pritchard FE, Minard G, Kudsk KA. A prospective analysis of diagnostic laparoscopy in trauma. Ann Surg 1993;217(5):557–564.

Case perspectives: Dan Schoenberger

THERAPEUTIC PERSPECTIVES

1 Shock

Shock is defined as 'inadequate tissue perfusion' and can be classified by its cause:

- Hypovolaemic
- Cardiogenic
- Septic
- Neurogenic
- Anaphylactic

Table 2 in the previous discussion defines the classification of shock along with its signs and symptoms.

DAN AND SHOCK

Dan is in stage 2 shock, but his BP is mildly low which puts him at the border of stage 3. He rapidly responds and if you reassessed him later you would see that his vital signs have returned to normal. Combined with the clinical scenario and blood results, this is a picture of dehydration resulting in hypovolaemia. However, in the postoperative setting it is important to rule out bleeding. Reviewing a patient gives a snapshot of their condition. If you intervene and make a change, you must monitor the result.

2 Inotropes

- Inotropes are agents which alter the energy of muscular contraction.
- They can be positive (increasing the energy of contraction) or negative (decreasing the energy of contraction) (Table 6 gives some common examples of each).

Table 6 Examples of positive and negative inotropes

Positive inotropes	Negative inotropes
Calcium	Beta-blockers
Digoxin	Calcium channel blockers
Catecholamines (e.g. adrenaline, noradrenaline, dopamine, dobutamine)	Antiarrhythmics (e.g. procainamide, flecainide)

*please refer to the Definitions at the end of this Case perspective.

- In the setting of intensive care and shock, the most commonly used inotropes are the catecholamines.
- Volume filling is the most important step in hypovolaemic shock.
- Adequate filling can be assessed with the help of central venous pressure (discussed below).
- Noradrenaline causes a peripheral vasoconstriction, thus increasing peripheral resistance and raising blod pressure.
- Noradrenaline can produce excessive vasoconstriction, resulting in impaired organ perfusion, peripheral ischaemia and increased afterload.
- This peripheral ischaemia has been implicated in the development of symmetrical peripheral gangrene.[1]
- Furthermore, the increased afterload can increase the workload of the myocardium.

DAN AND NORADRENALINE

Dan has inadequate volume to maintain his blood pressure and urine output. The noradrenaline will cause his blood pressure to rise and when this is above a critical point, urine output may improve. However, Dan does not have an adequate volume to maintain blood pressure and is likely to require an increasing volume of noradrenaline so that it remains effective. This can expose Dan to peripheral ischaemia and the increase in afterload mentioned above.

3 Central venous pressure

Central venous pressure is the pressure within one of the large veins in the thorax. It approximates to 'filling pressure of the right ventricle'. It allows estimation of the systemic 'preload'.

There are many things that interfere with CVP monitoring including catheter obstruction, incorrect calibration, incorrect tip position and PEEP.*

The change in CVP in response to a fluid challenge is far more important than the absolute value, and it should always be interpreted in conjunction with the clincial picture. For example, the hypovolaemic patient will initially respond to fluid with little or no change to CVP (e.g. 4 cmH$_2$O to 5 cmH$_2$O). In contrast, the overloaded patient will exhibit an abrupt and sustained rise in CVP (13 cmH$_2$O to 20 cmH$_2$O).

DAN AND CVP

Dan's CVP read 12 cmH$_2$O at the end of his surgery and now it reads 4 cmH$_2$O. If you challenged him with a fluid bolus, his CVP rose slightly to 6 cmH$_2$O, indicating that this was a hypovolaemic problem.

4 Transfusion of packed red blood cells (PRBC) in the intensive care unit

- The storage of PRBC reduces 2,3-diphosphoglycerate, thus increasing oxygen affinity and decreasing the ability of haemoglobin to offload oxygen.
- Morphological changes in stored erythrocytes may result in increased fragility and decreased viability of the cells.
- Transfusion of PRBC may increase the risk of the development of multi-organ failure.[2]
- The transfusion of PRBC containing leukocytes has immunomodulatory* effects.[3]
- Evidence has shown that postoperative patients who are transfused run a greater risk of bacterial infection than those elective patients who never receive a transfusion.[4]
- Transfusions have been shown to result in increased mortality and infection rates in burns patients.[5]
- Although the methodology of many of the studies has been criticised, a large volume of evidence suggests that blood transfusions may have a deleterious effect on patients. Many centres now recommend not transfusing unless the patient is haemodynamically unstable or has a Hb <7 g/dL. Although controversial, this has been shown to be safe.[6]

DAN AND BLOOD TRANSFUSION

Regardless of the points above regarding transfusion in the ICU, Dan has a Hb of 14.2 g/dL and based on this does not require transfusion. Although a drop in Hb can take time to occur following blood loss, the overall picture with an increase in HCT points to a concentrated specimen. Transfusing in this setting is at best a waste of resources and at worst potentially harmful to your patient. If you opted to transfuse, the haematologist would have refused and you would have been deducted points.

5 Urine output

- Urine output can act as a guide to monitor renal blood flow and thus as a guide to fluid resuscitation.
- Adequate volume in an adult should produce a urinary output of roughly 0.5 ml/kg/h, thus 35 ml/h in a 70 kg adult.
- Urinary output can be affected by other factors such as diruetics.

DAN AND URINE OUTPUT

When you find Dan, he has a urine output of just 12 ml/h. After administering fluid, it rises to 30 ml/h. If you did not reassess Dan after administering fluid, you would have rounded with Cahoon the following morning to find that his urine output had fallen again to 8 ml/h.

6 Biochemical markers of dehydration: urea/HCT/urinary specific gravity

- Urea
  - Produced by the liver as a waste product from the metabolism of protein.
  - Cleared in the kidneys.
  - Dehydration results in a rise in urea but not creatinine.
  - The rise in urea is an adaptive response by the loop of Henle and medullary collecting duct to potentiate the effect of vasopressin,* thus allowing for the greater retention of water from the filtrate.[7]
- Haematocrit
  - The ratio of the volume occupied by PRBC to the volume of the whole blood.
  - Normal range is males 40–52%, females 36–48%.
  - A raised HCT can result from a decrease in plasma volume (e.g. dehydration) or a rise in red cell mass (primary, e.g. polycythaemia, or secondary, e.g. smoking).
  - Genuine increased red cell mass is suspected when the HCT is >60% in males and >56% in females.
- Urinary specific gravity
  - The specific gravity of urine is the concentration of metabolites excreted in urine.
  - Normal specific gravity values range from 1.002 to 1.028 g/ml.
  - Specific gravity changes according to clinical presentation (Table 7).

Table 7 Causes of changes in specific gravity

>1.028 g/ml	<1.002 g/ml
Dehydration	Renal failure
Glucosuria	Pyelonephritis
Shock	Diabetes insipidus
	Acute tubular necrosis
	Interstitial nephritis
	Excessive fluid intake

DAN AND BIOCHEMICAL MARKERS OF DEHYDRATION

Dan has a urea of 13.1 and a normal creatinine, in keeping with dehydration. He also has a HCT of 57% which is high but not greater than 60%, which may point towards a true increase in red cell mass as the cause.

Furthermore, his urine has a specific gravity of 1.034 in keeping with a picture of dehyration and shock. Note: his sodium is marginally raised, reflecting a concentrated sample, as are his WBC. The WBC may also, as with the high CRP, be an inflammatory response from the surgery.

COMMUNICATION PERSPECTIVES

Intern's perspective

SIMPSON AND MIA CHANG

As you have encountered before, this is Mia's first night on call and she is naturally going to be a little anxious. It is your professional responsibility to help and be supportive where possible. If this were not reason enough, spending more time early on with your junior doctors will result in them learning more and training more quickly. Ultimately, this results in them being able to handle a broader range of clinical problems on their own.

What happened to Dan?

Dan made a good recovery. He left the ICU the following day and was discharged 5 days later. His histopathology report indicated a Dukes B tumour with good margins. As a result, he did not require postoperative chemotherapy.

DEFINITIONS

PEEP – positive end expiratory pressure. Pressure applied during expiration in patients on mechanical ventilation. This helps to keep the lungs from collapsing (atelectasis).

Immunomodulation – a factor which influences the working of the immune system.

Vasopressin – a hormone produced by the hypothalamus and stored in the posterior pituitary. It reduces water excretion by the kidenys and increases blood pressure by causing vasoconstriction.

REFERENCE LIST

1. Hayes MA, Yau EH, Hinds CJ, Watson JD. Symmetrical peripheral gangrene: association with noradrenaline administration. Intens Care Med 1992;18(7):433–436.
2. Zallen G, Offner PJ, Moore EE, et al. Age of transfused blood is an independent risk factor for postinjury multiple organ failure. Am J Surg 1999;178(6):570–572.
3. Blajchman MA. Transfusion immunomodulation or TRIM: what does it mean clinically? Hematology 2005;10(Suppl 1):208–214.

4. Hill GE, Frawley WH, Griffith KE, Forestner JE, Minei JP. Allogeneic blood transfusion increases the risk of postoperative bacterial infection: a meta-analysis. J Trauma 2003;54(5):908–914.

5. Palmieri TL, Caruso DM, Foster KN, et al. Effect of blood transfusion on outcome after major burn injury: a multicenter study. Crit Care Med 2006;34(6):1602–1607.

6. Earley AS, Gracias VH, Haut E, et al. Anemia management program reduces transfusion volumes, incidence of ventilator-associated pneumonia, and cost in trauma patients. J Trauma 2006;61(1):1–5.

7. Mehta AR. Why does the plasma urea concentration increase in acute dehydration? Adv Physiol Educ 2008;32(4):336.

INVESTIGATIONS

Name: Karen Twentyman
Adress: 2 Melview Heights
        Lower East Park
Specimen No: PH763517   (Haematology)

MRN: 109678   DOB: 29/09/1996
Loc: Emergency Dept. Pilgrims
Sex: F   Phone: Req by: Simpson
\<PgDn\> for later samples

PH763517   12/03/2011   20:37   Whole Blood

WBC	9.9	×10^9/L	(4 to 11) Auth
RBC	4.51	×10^12/l	(4.5 to 5.3) Auth
HB	14.2	g/dl	(12 to 16) Auth
HCT	0.40	l/l	(0.36 to 0.5) Auth
MCV	90.5	fl	(76 to 96) Auth
MCH	31.0	pg	(27 to 32) Auth
MCHC	34.3	g/dl	(32 to 36) Auth
PLT	224	×10^9/l	(140 to 440) Auth
Neutrophils	7.80	×10^9/l	(1.8 to 8) Auth
Lymphocytes	2.30	×10^9/l	(1.5 to 3.5) Auth
Monocytes	0.24	×10^9/l	(0.16 to 1) Auth
Eosinophils	0.16	×10^9/l	(0 to 0.5) Auth
Basophils	0.01	×10^9/l	(0 to 0.2) Auth
INR	1.1		(1 to 1.2) Auth
APTT	24	SEC	(22 to 30) Auth

1 Date   2 Earlst   3 Latst   4 rep seQ   5 Spec   6 DFT   7 Matches   8 Options   9 Exit X
No more samples
Disc: HAEM   Sect. Haem   Pilgrims Emergency department   WRNQ/APEX   Overtype

---

Name: Karen Twentyman
Adress: 2 Melview Heights
        Lower East Park
Specimen No: PH763517   (Biochemistry)

MRN: 109678   DOB: 29/09/1996
Loc: Emergency Dept. Pilgrims
Sex: F   Phone: Req by: Simpson
\<PgDn\> for later samples

PH763517   12/03/2011   20:37   Whole Blood

Sodium	142	mmol/L	(132 to 144) Auth
Potassium	4.2	mmol/L	(3.5 to 5.0) Auth
Chloride	91	mmol/L	(95 to 107) Auth
Urea	7.0	mmol/L	(2.5 to 7.0) Auth
Creatinine	70	umol/L	(50 to 130) Auth
Total Protein	64	g/L	(62 to 82) Auth
Albumin	40	g/L	(36 to 44) Auth
AST	38	U/L	(6 to 42) Auth
ALT	40	U/L	(4 to 45) Auth
Total Bilirubin	10	umol/L	(2 to 20) Auth
GGT	40	U/L	(6 to 48) Auth
Alkaline Phosphatase	100	U/L	(40 to 130) Auth
Amylase	54	U/L	(28 to 150) Auth
C-Reactive Protein	2	mg/L	(0 to 10) Auth
Calcium	2.4	mmol/L	(2.1 to 2.62) Auth
Haemolysis index	0		

1 Date   2 Earlst   3 Latst   4 rep seQ   5 Spec   6 DFT   7 Matches   8 Options   9 Exit X
Disc: Biochem   Sect: Biochem   Pilgrims Emergency department   WRNQ/APEX
Overtype

Name: Karen Twentyman   MRN: 109678   DOB: 29/09/1996
Adress: 2 Melview Heights   Loc: Emergency Dept. Pilgrims
        Lower East Park   Sex: F   Phone: Req by: Simpson
Specimen No: PH763517   (Biochemistry)   <PgDn> for later samples

PH763517	12/03/2011	20:37	Urinalysis Dipstick		
Colour	Yellow				Auth
Glucose	Negative		(	Negative	) Auth
Bilirubin	Negative		(	Negative	) Auth
Ketones	Positive 2+		(	Negative	) Auth
Specific Gravity	1.020		(1.014 to 1.028)		Auth
Blood	Negative		(	Negative	) Auth
pH	6.5		(	4.3 to 7.5	) Auth
Proteins	Negative	g/L	(	Negative	) Auth
Urobilinogen	16	umol/			Auth
Nitrate	Negative		(	Negative	) Auth
Leukocytes	Negative		(	Negative	) Auth

1 Date 2 Earlst 3 Latst 4 rep seQ 5 Spec 6 DFT 7 Matches 8 Options 9 Exit X
                           No Further Samples
Disc: Biochem Sect: Biochem Pilgrims Emergency department WRNQ/APEX
Overtype

Name: Sharyn Romanowska   MRN: 109680   DOB: 07/02/1949
Adress: 5 River Walk   Loc: Emergency Dept. Pilgrims
        Bayside   Sex: F   Phone: Req by: Simpson
Specimen No: PH763519   (Haematology)   <PgDn> for later samples

PH763517	12/03/2011	20:37	Whole Blood		
WBC	18.2	×10^9/L	(	4 to 11	) Auth
RBC	4.51	×10^12/l	(	4.5 to 5.3	) Auth
HB	14.2	g/dl	(	12 to 16	) Auth
HCT	0.53	l/l	(	0.36 to 0.5	) Auth
MCV	90.5	fl	(	76 to 96	) Auth
MCH	31.0	pg	(	27 to 32	) Auth
MCHC	34.3	g/dl	(	32 to 36	) Auth
PLT	520	×10^9/l	(	140 to 440	) Auth
Neutrophils	14.34	×10^9/l	(	1.8 to 8	) Auth
Lymphocytes	2.30	×10^9/l	(	1.5 to 3.5	) Auth
Monocytes	0.24	×10^9/l	(	0.16 to 1	) Auth
Eosinophils	0.16	×10^9/l	(	0 to 0.5	) Auth
Basophils	0.01	×10^9/l	(	0 to 0.2	) Auth
INR	1.1		(	1 to 1.2	) Auth
APTT	24	SEC	(	22 to 30	) Auth

1 Date 2 Earlst 3 Latst 4 rep seQ 5 Spec 6 DFT 7 Matches 8 Options 9 Exit X
                           No more samples
Disc: HAEM Sect: Haem Pilgrims Emergency department WRNQ/APEX Overtype

---

TRUST LIBRARY
TORBAY HOSPITAL TQ2 7AA

Name: Sharyn Romanowska   MRN: 109680   DOB: 07/02/1949
Adress: 5 River Walk   Loc: Emergency Dept. Pilgrims
    Bayside   Sex: F   Phone: Req by: Simpson
Specimen No: PH763517   (Biochemistry)   <PgDn> for later samples

PH763517	12/03/2011 20:37	Whole Blood		
Sodium	146	mmol/L	(132 to 144	) Auth
Potassium	3.6	mmol/L	(3.5 to 5.0	) Auth
Chloride	91	mmol/L	(95 to 107	) Auth
Urea	16.0	mmol/L	(2.5 to 7.0	) Auth
Creatinine	140	umol/L	(50 to 130	) Auth
Total Protein	64	g/L	(62 to 82	) Auth
Albumin	40	g/L	(36 to 44	) Auth
AST	38	U/L	(6 to 42	) Auth
ALT	40	U/L	(4 to 45	) Auth
Total Bilirubin	19	umol/L	(2 to 20	) Auth
GGT	40	U/L	(6 to 48	) Auth
Alkaline Phosphatase	100	U/L	(40 to 130	) Auth
Amylase	54	U/L	(28 to 150	) Auth
C-Reactive Protein	186	mg/L	(0 to 10	) Auth
Calcium	2.4	mmol/L	(2.1 to 2.62	) Auth
Haemolysis index	0			

1 Date 2 Earlst 3 Latst 4 rep seQ 5 Spec 6 DFT 7 Matches 8 Options 9 Exit X
Disc: Biochem Sect: Biochem Pilgrims Emergency department WRNQ/APEX
Overtype

Name: Dan Schoenberger   MRN: 109679   DOB: 2/03/1957
Adress: Apt 513 Hilltop   Loc: ICU Pilgrims
    Open Street   Sex: M   Phone: Req by: Simpson
Specimen No: PH763518   (Haematology)   <PgDn> for later samples

PH763517	12/03/2011 20:37	Whole Blood		
WBC	12.1	×10^9/L	(4 to 11	) Auth
RBC	4.51	×10^12/l	(4.5 to 5.3	) Auth
HB	14.2	g/dl	(12 to 16	) Auth
HCT	0.57	l/l	(0.36 to 0.5	) Auth
MCV	90.5	fl	(76 to 96	) Auth
MCH	31.0	pg	(27 to 32	) Auth
MCHC	34.3	g/dl	(32 to 36	) Auth
PLT	224	×10^9/l	(140 to 440	) Auth
Neutrophils	7.80	×10^9/l	(1.8 to 8	) Auth
Lymphocytes	2.30	×10^9/l	(1.5 to 3.5	) Auth
Monocytes	0.24	×10^9/l	(0.16 to 1	) Auth
Eosinophils	0.16	×10^9/l	(0 to 0.5	) Auth
Basophils	0.01	×10^9/l	(0 to 0.2	) Auth
INR	1.1		(1 to 1.2	) Auth
APTT	24	SEC	(22 to 30	) Auth

1 Date 2 Earlst 3 Latst 4 rep seQ 5 Spec 6 DFT 7 Matches 8 Options 9 Exit X
No more samples
Disc: HAEM Sect: Haem Pilgrims Emergency department WRNQ/APEX Overtype

Name: Dan Schoenberger   MRN: 109679   DOB: 02/03/1957
Adress: Apt 513 Hilltop   Loc: ICU Pilgrims
       Open Street   Sex: M   Phone: Req by: Simpson
Specimen No: PH763518   (Biochemistry)   <PgDn> for later samples

PH763517	12/03/2011 20:37	Whole Blood		
Sodium	145	mmol/L	(132 to 144)	Auth
Potassium	4.2	mmol/L	(3.5 to 5.0)	Auth
Chloride	91	mmol/L	(95 to 107)	Auth
Urea	13.1	mmol/L	(2.5 to 7.0)	Auth
Creatinine	70	umol/L	(50 to 130)	Auth
Total Protein	64	g/L	(62 to 82)	Auth
Albumin	40	g/L	(36 to 44)	Auth
AST	38	U/L	(6 to 42)	Auth
ALT	40	U/L	(4 to 45)	Auth
Total Bilirubin	10	umol/L	(2 to 20)	Auth
GGT	40	U/L	(6 to 48)	Auth
Alkaline Phosphatase	100	U/L	(40 to 130)	Auth
Amylase	54	U/L	(28 to 150)	Auth
C-Reactive Protein	45	mg/L	(0 to 10)	Auth
Calcium	2.4	mmol/L	(2.1 to 2.62)	Auth
Haemolysis index	0			

1 Date 2 Earlst 3 Latst 4 rep seQ 5 Spec 6 DFT 7 Matches 8 Options 9 Exit X
Disc: Biochem Sect: Biochem Pilgrims Emergency department WRNQ/APEX
Overtype

Name: Dan Schoenberger   MRN: 109679   DOB: 02/03/1957
Adress: Apt 513 Hilltop   Loc: ICU Pilgrims
       Open Street   Sex: M   Phone: Req by: Simpson
Specimen No: PH763518   (Biochemistry)   <PgDn> for later samples

PH763517	12/03/2011 20:37	Urinalysis Dipstick		
Colour	Dark Yellow			Auth
Glucose	Negative		(Negative)	Auth
Bilirubin	Negative		(Negative)	Auth
Ketones	Positive 1+		(Negative)	Auth
Specific Gravity	1.034		(1.014 to 1.028)	Auth
Blood	Negative		(Negative)	Auth
pH	6.5		(4.8 to 7.5)	Auth
Proteins	Negative	g/L	(Negative)	Auth
Urobilinogen	13	umol/		Auth
Nitrate	Negative		(Negative)	Auth
Leukocytes	Negative		(Negative)	Auth

1 Date 2 Earlst 3 Latst 4 rep seQ 5 Spec 6 DFT 7 Matches 8 Options 9 Exit X
                    No Further Samples
Disc: Biochem Sect: Biochem Pilgrims Emergency department WRNQ/APEX
Overtype

SECTION 2

What you're going to learn

After this section you will be able to manage the preoperative and postoperative patient.

What you might also learn

Following completion of this section, you will be capable of performing the following in an evidence-based fashion.

- Manage a GI bleed.
- Independently assess and manage patients referred from other healthcare professionals.
- Prescribe antibiotics in a safe manner and only when indicated.
- Effectively manage postoperative complications.
- Implement a preoperative risk reduction strategy.
- Manage non-operative peritonitis.
- Decide on the appropriate operative and non-operative management of patients seen in the emergency department.

22.20 BACK TO WORK

Having finished a cold pizza slice and leaving a half cup of black coffee, you ignore the 24-hour weather report on the news channel and head back down the stairs to the pit. It's getting late now and there's always a lull between when the sober go home and the drunks come in. Although there are still about 15 people in the waiting room, nobody's talking; instead they gaze mindlessly at the weather report you have just left, all hoping to get home before the sun comes up again. Like you've been working here for years rather than hours, nobody notices as you walk over to the surgical slot again. This time there's only one chart in the slot as the man with cellulitis has not reappeared. You take the chart and walk over to cubicle 12. Pulling back the curtain, you introduce yourself to a 73-year-old lady, Norma Nowak, who is sitting with her leg exposed, demonstrating an ulcer on her medial malleolus. She is a non-smoker and has known varicose veins. As you enter, her daughter stands up and offers to leave. Do you:

I. Politely ask her to leave ⤑ **289**

II. Tell her she is welcome to stay ⤑ **210**

III. Ask Norma if she would like her daughter to stay ⤑ **195**

166 Given her cardiac murmur, do you want to cover her with antibiotics?

I. Yes ⤑ **262**

II. No ⤑ **327**

167 You ring Cahoon, who comes down to see the patient and agrees that it is a difficult case, particularly given Regina's cardiac status and the possibility of her requiring an anaesthetic. Ruth proceeds to try thrombolysis and eventually her efforts are successful and gradually over several hours Regina's leg becomes reperfused. Will you keep her anticoagulated?

I. Yes ⤑ **293**

II. No ⤑ **263**

168 There are no gallstones in the gallbladder, but it is difficult to see the pancreas as it is obscured by gas-filled loops of bowel. What would you like to do next?

I. Order a CXR ⤑ **190**

II. Order a CT abdomen ⤑ **205**

III. Start antibiotics and order a CT abdomen ⤑ **203**

IV. Start antibiotics ⤑ **304**

169 Satisfied at your explanation that she needs no further follow-up, Susie leaves the department to catch the end of her evening ball. In about 8 months she will return to the intensive care unit with gallstone pancreatitis. **Deduct 1 point**. You return to the slot and pick up the chart of your next patient.

⤑ **279**

170 You see a shallow ulcer over her medial malleolus, with no erythema and some slough at the base. **Deduct 1 point**. Take a history

⤑ **260**

171 You hold off on the nitrates; **add 1 point**. Do you want to give morphine?

I. Yes ⤑ **312**

II. No ⤑ **188**

172 You phone Cahoon and let him know your plan to perform an endoscopy. **Add 1 point.** He is very impressed and lets you do the endoscopy. Twenty minutes later you are passing the camera into Una's stomach. Inside you find copious amounts of black altered blood. You suck and irrigate at Cahoon's instructions. However, you do not see any ulcer or bleeding point. Just as Cahoon instructs you to check the duodenum, his bleep goes off. He tells you to carry on and he'll be back in a minute. You pass the scope into the first part of her duodenum and you see a large ulcer in the bulb of her duodenum. It is actively oozing, so you ask the nurse to get Cahoon but she returns to tell you she cannot find him. What do you want to do?

　I. Wait ⸱⸱⸱⟫ **257**

　II. Inject the ulcer ⸱⸱⸱⟫ **286**

　III. Withdraw and report to Cahoon what you have found ⸱⸱⸱⟫ **253**

173 The nurse passes you the endoscopic needle loaded with saline. Where would you like to inject?

　I. Just inferior to the ulcer ⸱⸱⸱⟫ **243**

　II. Into the bleeding point in the centre of the ulcer ⸱⸱⸱⟫ **189**

174 You ask Ruth to hold off on draining the cyst for now, and Marco is returned to the emergency department to await a bed. **Add 1 point.** How do you plan to predict his outcome over the next few days?

　I. Modified Glasgow (Imrie) criteria ⸱⸱⸱⟫ **254**

　II. Serial CRPs ⸱⸱⸱⟫ **292**

　III. Ranson's criteria ⸱⸱⸱⟫ **179**

175 Good, your suspicion is that of gallstones; **add 1 point.** Ruth happens to be in the department and does the scan immediately for you. It demonstrates multiple gallstones, a normal calibre common bile duct, no thickened gallbladder wall or fluid. What will you do next?

　I. Allow her home but bring her back to the clinic ⸱⸱⸱⟫ **285**

　II. Allow her home but don't bring her back so as not to clog up the outpatients ⸱⸱⸱⟫ **169**

　III. Tell her that she needs to lose weight ⸱⸱⸱⟫ **288**

　IV. Schedule surgery as an outpatient, and allow her home ⸱⸱⸱⟫ **255**

176 Three hours later the swamped radiology department returns your x-ray. There is no evidence of osteomyelitis or abnormalities. **Deduct 2 points.** What will you do now?

> I. Admit for intravenous benzylpenicillin and flucloxacillin ⋯⟶ **318**

> II. Allow home with a non-constricting dressing and a course of penicillin and flucloxacillin ⋯⟶ **180**

> III. Replace the original tight dressings that the nurse removed and send the patient home to be followed up by her surgeon ⋯⟶ **232.**

> IV. Allow home, swab the ulcer and if positive prescribe a course of antibiotics appropriate to culture ⋯⟶ **256**

177 You hold off on starting a beta-blocker; **deduct 1 point**. Would you also like to give clopidogrel?

> I. Yes ⋯⟶ **275**

> II. No ⋯⟶ **237**

> III. Phone the cardiologist ⋯⟶ **218**

178 Marco lies down flat on the trolley; **deduct 1 point**. His pulse is 112, BP 110/82, temp 37.1°C and O_2 saturations are 92%. His tongue is fissured and dry, and he has involuntary guarding with localised rebound in his epigastric region. The rest of his abdomen is soft and non-tender. His blood results are available in the Investigations at the end of this section. What will you do next?

> I. Get a history ⋯⟶ **228**

> II. Give him IV fluids ⋯⟶ **242**

> III. Give supplemental oxygen ⋯⟶ **290**

> IV. Order radiology ⋯⟶ **198**

> V. Take him to theatre immediately ⋯⟶ **313**

179 Calculating Marco's Ranson's score at 24 hours, you see that he scores 2 for his WBC and AST.

> ⋯⟶ **213**

180 Norma and her daughter are very grateful for your help. However, several days later Halsted receives a phone call from her surgeon complaining that young nurses and doctors these days *'just wouldn't know a non-infected venous ulcer if it bit them. I'm sick of these kids throwing antibiotics around like sweets'*. Halsted apologises on your behalf; **deduct 1 point**.

> ⋯⟶ **183**

181 Susie leaves for the end of her ball with her date for surgery. She returns 5 weeks later for her laparoscopic cholecystectomy. Cahoon is carrying out the surgery but becomes irate when he sees that nobody has advised her to stop smoking, even for 4 weeks preoperatively. **Deduct 1 point** and keep your head down.

···⟩ **279**

182 You give him pethidine (merperidine) and within a minute or two he has settled back into the trolley and looks considerably more comfortable. Will you:

   I. Take a history ···⟩ **221**

   II. Examine him ···⟩ **178**

183 The department is getting busy and the medical team have eight charts waiting in their slot. You pick up the two charts in the surgical slot, glad you're not a physician. The first is a 34-year-old woman with right upper quadrant pain and the second is a 23-year-old man with epigastric pain and vomiting. What do you want to do?

   I. See the woman with right upper quadrant pain ···⟩ **276**

   II. See the man with vomiting and epigastric pain ···⟩ **297**

   III. Read more about each patient ···⟩ **231**

184 You call Cahoon but he is stuck in a difficult case and won't be free to talk for another 5 minutes. Do you:

   I. Ask Ruth to drain the cyst ···⟩ **244**

   II. Tell Ruth not to drain the cyst ···⟩ **174**

   III. Tell Ruth you'll call her back in 5 minutes when you've spoken to Cahoon ···⟩ **323**

185 You ring Ruth to order a CT. '*Surely, given that history you're looking for gallstones?*' she asks. Meekly you agree. '*Well, it's an ultrasound you need, not a CT. I'm down in the department now and I'll do it right away if you can get the patient up to me.*' **Deduct 1 point**. The ultrasound demonstrates multiple small gallstones, a normal calibre common bile duct, no thickened gallbladder wall or fluid. What will you do next?

   I. Allow her home but bring her back to the clinic ···⟩ **285**

   II. Allow her home and not bring her back in order to avoid overbooking the clinic ···⟩ **169**

III. Tell her to lose weight ⋯⟩ 288

IV. Schedule surgery and allow her home ⋯⟩ 255

186 Marco benefits from the supplemental oxygen and his O_2 saturations quickly rise to 98%. What will you do next?

I. Order radiology ⋯⟩ 198

II. Give antibiotics ⋯⟩ 235

187 Recognising that Una's symptoms and history amount to probable bleeding from peptic ulcer disease rather than varices, you choose correctly not to pass a Sengstaken tube and instead start a proton pump inhibitor. **Add 1 point**. Joy tells you that the lab is on the phone, and they want to know if you would like platelets for Una.

I. Yes ⋯⟩ 234

II. No ⋯⟩ 266

188 You hold off on the morphine; **add 1 point**. Would you like to start a beta-blocker?

I. Yes ⋯⟩ 200

II. No ⋯⟩ 177

189 Good, **add 1 point**. You inject approximately 2 ml into the bleeding point at the base of the ulcer. It blanches nicely and the bleeding stops. Cahoon returns looking hassled, but is very impressed. He slaps you on the back and says, *'Well, let's see how she gets on tonight. I have to go and help Halsted in theatre, I'll see you later'*. Delighted with the praise, you remove the scope. Regarding her proton pump inhibitor, the nurse would like to know if you want to:

I. Stop it ⋯⟩ 222

II. Leave it as a once-daily dose ⋯⟩ 280

III. Increase it to a twice-daily dose ⋯⟩ 241

IV. Start a continuous infusion ⋯⟩ 226

190 The chest x-ray shows a small pleural effusion on the right side. However, as Marco is comfortable now and saturating normally, you decide to observe it. What do you want to do next?

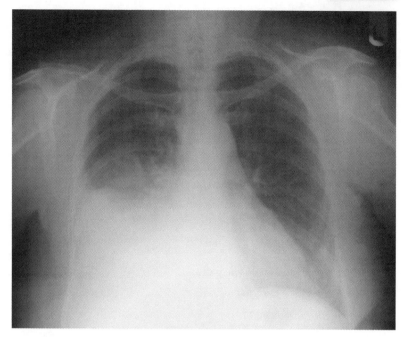

Chest x-ray of Marco Baldinelli.

I. Order a CT abdomen ⋯⟩ **205**

II. Start antibiotics and get a CT abdomen ⋯⟩ **203**

III. Start antibiotics ⋯⟩ **304**

191 You ask for 1:100,000 adrenaline and the nurse hands you the endoscopic needle. **Add 1 point**. Where would you like to inject?

I. Just inferior to the ulcer ⋯⟩ **243**

II. Into the bleeding point in the centre of the ulcer ⋯⟩ **189**

192 Ruth asks you the site of the patient's maximal tenderness. Unable to tell her, and caught unawares, you stutter. Impatiently, she says, *'Go and examine the patient and stop wasting my time,'* as she puts the phone down on you. **Deduct 1 point**.

⋯⟩ **298**

193 Marco is uncomfortable and hypertensive. Certainly, making him more comfortable should be a priority, and this will also help in getting good clinical details. **Add 1 point**. Would you like to give him:

I. Morphine ⋯⟩ **302**

II. Pethidine (merperidine) ⋯⟩ **182**

194 Nicola agrees to help you do an embolectomy under local anaesthetic and brings Regina to theatre. You call Cahoon and he joins you in theatre, performing an embolectomy under local anaesthetic. You fish some clot from the popliteal artery and her leg almost immediately pinks up and her dorsalis pedis pulse returns. Will you keep her anticoagulated?

> *I. Yes* ⋯⊱ **293**

> *II. No* ⋯⊱ **263**

195 Norma looks surprised but smiles and tells you that she would like her daughter to stay. *'I've an awful memory, doctor, I'll forget everything you tell me,'* she laughs. **Add 1 point**.

> *I. Examine her* ⋯⊱ **170**

> *II. Take a history* ⋯⊱ **225**

196 What type of aspirin do you give?

> *I. Enteric coated* ⋯⊱ **326**

> *II. Not enteric coated* ⋯⊱ **227**

197 The lady and her daughter are grateful for your attention; however, they are a little tired, as they have been in the emergency department for several hours now. **Deduct 1 point**. They thank you and leave. Wearily, you return to the surgical slot.

> ⋯⊱ **183**

198 What would you like to order?

> *I. Ultrasound* ⋯⊱ **168**

> *II. Chest x-ray* ⋯⊱ **271**

> *III. CT abdomen* ⋯⊱ **205**

199 You ring Cahoon and he agrees that a general anaesthetic would be dangerous and together you perform an embolectomy under local anaesthetic. **Add 1 point**. You fish a clot from her popliteal artery and almost immediately her leg pinks up and her dorsalis pedis pulse returns. Will you keep her anticoagulated?

> *I. Yes* ⋯⊱ **293**

> *II. No* ⋯⊱ **263**

200 You start a beta-blocker; **add 1 point**. Would you also like to give clopidogrel?

I. Yes ⇢ **275**

II. No ⇢ **237**

III. Phone the cardiologist ⇢ **218**

201 Marco mumbles incomprehensibly while Una tries to give you the story. Halfway through, Marco pushes over the trolley and, standing beside his bed, shouts, '*Do I not get anything for the pain, doc? This place is like a zoo*'. Hastily you draw up 10 mg of morphine and cyclizine and administer it IV. Within 3 minutes he has settled back into the bed as a security guard, aware of the tension, hovers nervously outside the curtain. Una gives most of the history with Marco adding pieces intermittently. It transpires that 4 weeks ago Marco won a sizeable amount of money on a horse race. He then booked a 2-week holiday in the sun, from which they have just both returned. From what Una tells you, there is nothing of the money left and it appears that they have spent nearly all of it on alcohol. The pain started suddenly before they left for the flight home and has become increasingly worse since. He has vomited several times but that seems to have eased now. Marco tells you that he is very thirsty but afraid that if he drinks he'll start to vomit again. You nod and tell him that you need to examine him.

⇢ **274**

202 You push on, ignoring Ubeki who rings Cahoon herself. Just as you're drawing up the urokinase, Cahoon comes in: '*What on earth are you doing, Simpson?*' he asks, taking the syringe from you. '*This lady is having a NSTEMI. I'm not a cardiologist but even I know you don't thrombolyse them. Listen, Simpson, I can't take it any more, go home and I'll talk to Halsted in the morning.*' Irritated, you throw your pen across the room, immediately knowing that it hasn't done you any good. Your shift is over.

203 Knowing that meropenem has the best pancreatic penetration, you draw it up and administer it intravenously. Happy that he is comfortable and stable and that his urine output is adequate, you explain the patient's case to Ruth and she agrees that a CT would help. The CT demonstrates reduced perfusion in about 20% of the pancreas with surrounding inflammation and some free fluid in the pelvis. In the body of the pancreas there is a 2 cm cyst. At the base of the right lung the CT has caught a small effusion. The whole picture certainly confirms that of an acute pancreatitis. Ruth rings you and asks if you want her to drain the cyst. Do you:

I. Say yes ⇢ **244**

II. Say no ⇢ **174**

III. Ring Cahoon and ask his advice ⇢ **184**

204 Three hours later the already swamped radiology department returns your x-ray. There is no evidence of osteomyelitis or abnormalities. **Deduct 1 point**.

> *I. Order a blood count, ESR and CRP* ⇢ **270**

> *II. Admit Norma for intravenous benzylpenicillin and flucloxacillin* ⇢ **318**

> *III. Allow Norma home with a non-constricting dressing and a course of penicillin and flucloxacillin* ⇢ **180**

> *IV. Allow Norma home, swab the ulcer and if positive prescribe a course of antibiotics appropriate to culture* ⇢ **256**

> *V. Replace the compression dressings that the nurse removed, reassure Norma and send her home to be followed up by her regular surgeon* ⇢ **232**

205 You explain Marco's case to Ruth and she agrees that a CT would help. The CT demonstrates reduced perfusion in about 20% of the pancreas with surrounding inflammation and some free fluid in the pelvis. In the body of the pancreas there is a 2 cm cyst. At the base of the right lung the CT shows a small effusion. The picture certainly confirms that of an acute pancreatitis. Ruth rings you and asks if you want her to drain the cyst. Do you:

> *I. Say yes* ⇢ **244**

> *II. Say no* ⇢ **174**

> *III. Ring Cahoon and ask his advice* ⇢ **184**

206 Ruth happens to be in the department and does the scan immediately for you. It demonstrates multiple gallstones, a normal calibre common bile duct, no thickened gallbladder wall or fluid. What will you do next?

> *I. Allow her home but bring her back to the clinic* ⇢ **285**

> *II. Allow her home and don't bring her back, trying to limit the amount of returns to the clinic* ⇢ **169**

> *III. Tell her to lose weight* ⇢ **288**

> *IV. Schedule surgery and allow her home* ⇢ **255**

207 Susie tells you that '*I'll just die without my cigarettes. I've tried but it's impossible for me to go more than 4 weeks without them*'. Do you:

> *I. Refuse her surgery and send her away* ⇢ **277**

> *II. Tell her to give up 3 weeks before surgery* ⇢ **291**

> *III. Smile and tell her not to worry about it* ⇢ **181**

208 What would you like to start?

   I. Unfractionated heparin (UH) ⋯⟩ **316**

   II. Low molecular weight heparin (LMWH) ⋯⟩ **267**

209 You gently take off the temporary dressing and there is a shallow ulcer over the medial malleolus. It has a little slough at the centre but is otherwise clean. She has strong dorsalis pedis and posterior tibial pulses. How will you manage Mrs Nowak?

   I. Order a blood count, ESR and CRP ⋯⟩ **300**

   II. Order an x-ray ⋯⟩ **204**

   III. Admit Norma for intravenous benzylpenicillin and flucloxacillin ⋯⟩ **318**

   IV. Allow Norma home with a non-constricting dressing and a course of penicillin and flucloxacillin ⋯⟩ **180**

   V. Replace the compression dressings that the nurse removed, reassure Norma and send her home to be followed up by her regular surgeon ⋯⟩ **232**

   VI. Allow home, swab the ulcer and if positive prescribe a course of antibiotics appropriate to culture ⋯⟩ **256**

210 The daughter thanks you and Norma smiles.

   I. Examine her ⋯⟩ **170**

   II. Take a history ⋯⟩ **225**

211 Given that Regina is going to need some form of intervention, you opt for UH and give a bolus before starting an infusion. You should have started this by now; **deduct 1 point**. What will you do next?

   I. Contact Nicola to arrange an embolectomy ⋯⟩ **295**

   II. Go to the radiology department and ask Ruth to use thrombolysis ⋯⟩ **233**

212 You have the result within 30 minutes and Ruth tells you that there is a clear cut-off at the left distal superficial femoral artery, suggesting an embolism. Do you want to:

   I. Start heparin ⋯⟩ **211**

   II. Ask Ruth to clear it with thrombolysis ⋯⟩ **233**

   III. Ring Nicola and organise an embolectomy ⋯⟩ **295**

Section 2

213 You follow Marco back to the department and, pulling back the curtain, you see him putting on his trousers and shirt. Una is behind him, pale and crying, pleading with him to stay. She looks up as you enter: '*Tell him to stay, doctor; please tell him to stay, he says he's going home*'. Will you:

> *I. Allow him to go* ⟶ **303**

> *II. Try to reason with him* ⟶ **219**

214 Una gags and becomes very distressed as you try to pass the Sengstaken–Blakemore tube down her oropharynx. She vomits twice as a result. Outside, Marco pushes the security guard away and shouts '*What's he doing to her?*'. Joy becomes worried and asks if she should call anybody to help. Impatiently you tell her to wait. In the interim Margaret has phoned Cahoon, who now arrives. You put the tube, now dripping with bloody mucus, down while you tell him the story and he tells you to put the tube away. '*Simpson, this doesn't sound remotely like oesophageal varices. She needs an upper endoscopy for a likely ulcer . . . well doesn't she?*' You shuffle awkwardly as he stares at you and then the tube. '*Look, just go and see somebody else and I'll take care of this lady*', he says. **Deduct 1 point**.

⟶ **299**

215 Susie leaves with her date for surgery. She returns 5 weeks later for her laparoscopic cholecystectomy. Cahoon is carrying out the surgery but becomes irate when he sees that nobody has advised her to stop smoking or stop her contraceptive pill. **Deduct 1 point** and keep your head down.

⟶ **279**

216 Susie looks at her watch impatiently. '*Listen, doc, I'm under pressure for time here.*' Slightly irritated but hiding it well, you call radiology. Although she is on the oral contraceptive pill, you double check that she is not pregnant with a urine sample. What would you like to request?

> *I. PFA* ⟶ **230**

> *II. Ultrasound abdomen* ⟶ **175**

> *III. CT abdomen* ⟶ **185**

217 OK, so you didn't score as well as we know you can. This might be because Cahoon sent you off early in a case or two. Don't worry, mistakes do happen and we all make bad choices. However, with books like this, websites and vignettes, it now means that we can make these mistakes without hurting patients. Make as many mistakes this way instead of where it counts. That way your patients will get the most from you. Martin Fischer, the German-American physician and writer, made a lot of sense when he said, *'The patient does not care about your science; what he wants to know is, can you cure him?'*. Maybe think about doing the section again, perhaps after you have done Section 3, and show yourself how much you have learned.

218 You ask the cardiologist who says to hold off as he is on his way to see the patient and will decide. **Add 1 point.**

···⟩ 305

219 Marco is visibly sweating while he dresses and it is clear that he is unwell and needs to stay. *'Listen, Marco,'* you start but he does not listen. *'You know what you can do, doc, don't you?'* he shouts. You try to reason. *'Marco, you're sick and we're just trying to help you.'* *'Well, you can shove it, doc, I'm leaving,'* he says, turning to Una. *'Well, are you coming or what?'* he asks her aggressively. His stare fixes on his girlfriend. *'Una?'* Una has become pale and she suddenly vomits about 500 ml of bright red blood onto the bed in the cubicle. Reacting quickly, you call for one of the nurses and put her onto the next trolley. Marco begins to shout as the security team arrives to investigate the commotion. You leave a nurse with Marco and wheel Una into the resuscitation room, wondering if tonight is ever going to end.

···⟩ 324

220 Mrs Nowak has no pain and generally feels well. She was never a smoker and is not a diabetic. She is sketchy on the details but apparently the ulcer has been there for a long time. How will you manage Mrs Nowak?

> I. *Order a blood count, ESR and CRP* ···⟩ **300**

> II. *Order an x-ray* ···⟩ **176**

> III. *Admit Norma for intravenous benzylpenicillin and flucloxacillin* ···⟩ **318**

> IV. *Allow Norma home with a non-constricting dressing and a course of oral penicillin and flucloxacillin* ···⟩ **180**

> V. *Allow Norma home, swab the ulcer and if positive prescribe a course of antibiotics appropriate to culture* ···⟩ **256**

> VI. *Replace the compression dressings that the nurse removed, reassure Norma and send her home to be followed up by her regular surgeon* ···⟩ **232**

221 Una gives most of the history with Marco adding pieces intermittently. It transpires that 4 weeks ago Marco won a small amount of money on a horse race. He then booked a 2-week holiday in the sun, from which they have both just returned. From what Una tells you, there is nothing of the money left and it appears that they have spent nearly all of it on alcohol. The pain started suddenly before they left for the flight home and has become increasingly worse since. He has vomited several times but that seems to have eased now. Marco tells you that he is very thirsty but is afraid that if he drinks he'll start to vomit again. You nod and tell him that you need to examine him.

⋯⟩ **274**

222 You discontinue the proton pump inhibitor now that the bleeding has stopped and you return to the slot. Tomorrow night Winston is on call and Una rebleeds. As they bring her to theatre, he has great satisfaction telling Cahoon that the whole mess was avoidable, but that 'somebody' stopped her proton pump inhibitor. Cahoon promises to 'look into it' as Winston hands him her chart, open on your note of course. **Deduct 1 point**.

⋯⟩ **299**

223 You run it by Cahoon who tells you that thrombolysis is a bad idea as there is no ST elevation. He does advise you to start heparin and contact the cardiologist to get advice on how to maximise her medical care.

⋯⟩ **321**

224 You advise her to stop her contraceptive pill before surgery and use alternative contraception, in order to reduce her risk of thrombosis. **Add 1 point**. Will you next:

I. *Tell her to stop smoking* ⋯⟩ **317**

II. *Allow her home and schedule surgery* ⋯⟩ **181**

225 With the help of her daughter, Mrs Nowak explains that she has had a leg ulcer for nearly a month. It has been looked after by a local surgeon who recently changed her to a tight dressing, which has helped enormously, with the ulcer reducing dramatically over the past 2 weeks. Today her normal nurse was away and she had a new nurse dress the wound. The new nurse was worried that the ulcer was infected and sent her to the emergency department. Mrs Nowak has no pain and generally feels well. She was never a smoker and is not a diabetic. '*I really think it's fine, doctor*' she tells you, smiling. **Add 1 point**. Would you like to:

I. *Examine her* ⋯⟩ **209**

II. *Order a full blood count, ESR and CRP* ⋯⟩ **300**

III. *Order an x-ray* ⋯⟩ **204**

226 Excellent work. **Add 1 point**. She has already been given a bolus of omeprazole and you now start an infusion. Over the next 24 hours Una settles completely and goes home 2 days later. She has a repeat endoscopy 4 weeks later which shows that the ulcer has completely healed. Well done.

⋯⟶ **299**

227 You give the non-enteric coated aspirin; **add 1 point**. Do you want to administer oxygen?

I. Yes ⋯⟶ **259**

II. No ⋯⟶ **309**

228 Una gives most of the history with Marco adding pieces intermittently. It transpires that 4 weeks ago Marco won a small amount of money on a horse race. He then booked a 2-week holiday in the sun, from which they have both just returned. From what Una tells you, there is nothing of the money left and it appears that they have spent nearly all of it on alcohol. The pain started suddenly before they left for the flight home and has become increasingly worse since. He has vomited several times but that seems to have eased now. Marco tells you that he is very thirsty but afraid that if he drinks he'll start to vomit again. What do you want to do next?

I. Give him IV fluids ⋯⟶ **242**

II. Give supplemental oxygen ⋯⟶ **290**

III. Order radiology ⋯⟶ **198**

IV. Take him to theatre immediately ⋯⟶ **313**

229 Superb. You don't need us to tell you that this is a great score. Maximum points are not easy. It means not putting a foot wrong, which is something that is nice to do but impossible to always maintain. At certain times we all make judgements that are far from perfect, so although you did well on Section 2, don't get too cocky. Confucius, the Chinese social philosopher, once said: *'By three methods we may learn wisdom: first by reflection which is the noblest, second by imitation which is the easiest and third by experience which is the bitterest'*. Books like this and the internet let you gain experience without it being as 'bitter' as real life, so use them as much as possible. Well done again on a perfect score in Section 2. Now get back to work in Section 3.

230 The PFA shows nothing; **deduct 1 point**. What would you like to do?

I. Ultrasound abdomen ⋯⟶ **206**

II. CT abdomen ⋯⟶ **185**

III. Allow her home but bring her back to the clinic ⋯⟶ **261**

Section 2

IV. Allow her home and don't bring her back in order to reduce the amount of returns to the clinic ⋯⟩ **169**

231 Good, it's always worthwhile reading the charts first to prioritise your patients. **Add 1 point**. The lady had one episode of right upper quadrant pain 5 hours ago, lasting 2 hours. She is pain free now and her pulse is 72, BP 110/64, O_2 saturations 100% and temperature normal. The man has just returned from holiday with severe epigastric pain and vomiting. His pulse is 112, BP is 178/98, O_2 saturations 90% and temperature is normal. Do you:

I. See the woman ⋯⟩ **311**

II. See the man ⋯⟩ **287**

232 Superb. You confidently reassure the patient that her ulcer is not infected and that the compression bandaging is certainly working. Delighted, both Norma and her daughter go home promptly. Several days later Halsted hands you a thank you card that arrived to his office for you from Mrs Nowak's daughter. *'Well done'* grunts Halsted. **Add 1 point**.

⋯⟩ **183**

233 Do you want to use:

I. Localised thrombolysis ⋯⟩ **325**

II. Systemic thrombolysis ⋯⟩ **306**

234 Despite Una's platelets being normal and the fact that she is not on any antiplatelet medications, you order two pools of precious platelets. **Deduct 1 point**. Her tachycardia is now 104. Do you want to perform an upper endoscopy?

I. Yes ⋯⟩ **166**

II. No ⋯⟩ **265**

235 Knowing that meropenem has the best pancreatic penetration, you draw it up and administer it intravenously. Happy that he is comfortable and stable and that his urine output is adequate, you decide to investigate further with radiology.

⋯⟩ **198**

236 You see a shallow ulcer, with no erythema and some slough at the base. **Deduct 1 point**. Take a history.

⋯⟩ **220**

237 You hold off on adding a loading does of clopidogrel.

⋯⟩ **305**

238 Recognising from this man's signs, symptoms and bloods that he has a likely pancreatitis, you need to fluid resuscitate him aggressively while monitoring his urine output. Do you:

> *I. Give 500 ml over 1 hour and titrate more fluid to his hourly urine output* ⋯⟩ **308**

> *II. Give 2 litres stat followed by 1 litre over 2 hours and then titrate to his hourly urine output* ⋯⟩ **249**

239 Given the recent surgery, you decide not to give 300 mg aspirin. **Deduct 1 point**. It certainly seems that she has had a cardiac ischaemic event. Do you want to thrombolyse her?

> *I. Yes* ⋯⟩ **281**

> *II. No* ⋯⟩ **296**

240 Well done, this is a good score. You've obviously managed to work your way through most of the cases successfully while minimising the negative marks. Your core knowledge is important and as William Osler, the legendary clinician, once said, '*The greater the ignorance, the greater the dogmatism*'. However, equally important is your ability to read a situation and read people. The former comes with study, the latter with experience. Well done, now see how you do in the final section.

241 You increase her proton pump inhibitor to a twice-daily dose. Over the next 48 hours she settles and is then allowed home. Four weeks later she has a repeat endoscopy which demonstrates a healed ulcer. Right now, happy with yourself, you return to the surgical slot.

> ⋯⟩ **299**

242 Recognising from this man's signs, symptoms and bloods that he has a likely pancreatitis, you need to fluid resuscitate him aggressively while monitoring his urine output. Do you:

> *I. Give 500 ml over 1 hour and then titrate further fluid to his hourly urine output* ⋯⟩ **308**

> *II. Give 2 litres stat followed by 1 litre over 2 hours and then titrate to his hourly urine output* ⋯⟩ **268**

243 You inject just inferior to the ulcer, but it does nothing to arrest the bleeding. Just then Cahoon returns. '*Well, what have you found, Simpson?*' he asks. '*You need to inject the bleeding point in the ulcer,*' he explains. You follow his advice, causing the bleeding to tamponade. '*Well done,*' he tells you. '*I need to go and help Halsted in theatre. I'll talk to you later.*' Pleased with his praise, would you next like to:

I. *Stop her proton pump inhibitor* ⋯⟫ **222**

II. *Leave her proton pump inhibitor as a once-daily dose* ⋯⟫ **280**

III. *Increase her proton pump inhibitor to a twice-daily dose* ⋯⟫ **241**

IV. *Start a continuous infusion of a proton pump inhibitor* ⋯⟫ **226**

244 Under CT guidance Ruth tries to drain the small cyst, removing just 1.5 ml of straw-coloured fluid. Disappointed with herself, she tells you she can't get any more out and is going home. **Deduct 1 point**. Marco is returned to the emergency department where you head to meet him.

⋯⟫ **273**

245 Marco sits back slowly, groaning. **Deduct 1 point**. He mumbles incomprehensibly while Una tries to give you the story. Halfway through, Marco gets up and pushes over the trolley beside his bed, shouting *'Do I not get anything for the pain, doc? This place is like a zoo'*. You hastily administer 10 mg morphine with cyclizine and within 3 minutes his pain settles. Marco lies down flat on the trolley. His pulse is 112, BP 110/82, temp 37.1°C and O_2 saturations 92%. His tongue is fissured and dry and he has involuntary guarding with localised rebound in his epigastric region. The rest of his abdomen is soft and non-tender. His blood results are available in the Investigations at the end of this section. What will you do next?

I. *Get a history* ⋯⟫ **228**

II. *Give him IV fluids* ⋯⟫ **242**

III. *Give supplemental oxygen* ⋯⟫ **290**

IV. *Order radiology* ⋯⟫ **198**

V. *Take him to theatre immediately* ⋯⟫ **313**

246 You group and save, wanting to conserve blood as much as possible. However, 15 minutes later she vomits again, mostly coffee grounds but there are some flecks of bright red blood. Her pulse is now 108 and her BP is 100/70. You ring the lab and cross-match her for two units. Do you want to pass a Sengstaken–Blakemore tube?

I. *Yes* ⋯⟫ **214**

II. *No* ⋯⟫ **187**

247 Pulling back the curtain, you meet Susie Redback, a 34-year-old teacher. She is sitting on the chair beside the bed and smiles when you walk in. She developed a sudden-onset right upper quadrant pain about 4 hours ago. It radiated to her right shoulder and lasted about 30 minutes. Although quite severe at the time, causing her to vomit once, it is entirely gone now. Previously she has had 'twinges' of pain but not as severe as this. She smokes 10 cigarettes per day and the only medication she takes is the oral contraceptive pill. Her bloods are available in the Investigations at the end of this section. What would you like to do next?

> *I. Examine her* ⇢ **298**

> *II. Order radiology* ⇢ **192**

248 You administer sublingual nitrates; **deduct 1 point**. Do you want to give morphine next?

> *I. Yes* ⇢ **312**

> *II. No* ⇢ **188**

249 Good. Although he does not make any urine initially, by the third litre he is putting out 25 ml per hour. **Add 1 point**. Happy that he has also had enough analgesia, what will you do next?

> *I. Order radiology* ⇢ **198**

> *II. Give antibiotics* ⇢ **235**

250 Norma has no pain and generally feels well. She was never a smoker and is not a diabetic. She is sketchy on the details and more interested in asking you where you are from, but apparently the ulcer has been there for a long time. Examine her.

> ⇢ **209**

251 You contact radiology and organise a lower limb angiogram. By the time it has been performed and reported, a further hour has passed. Ruth tells you that there is a clear cut-off point at the left distal superficial femoral artery, in keeping with the appearance of an acute embolus. Do you:

> *I. Contact Nicola, your anaesthetist, and organise an embolectomy* ⇢ **295**

> *II. Use thrombolysis* ⇢ **233**

252 You pull back the curtain and Marco Baldinelli is leaning forward holding his epigastrium. Una Lordan, his girlfriend, is rubbing his back as you enter and they both look up. You introduce yourself and he grunts incomprehensibly at you. Una apologises and explains that he has been up all night with pain. You nod consolingly and tell them that you understand completely, while deep down you know this is going to be an awkward one. Do you:

I. Take a history ⋯⟩ **201**

II. Ask him to sit back, and examine him ⋯⟩ **245**

III. Give analgesia ⋯⟩ **193**

253 You remove the scope and just as you're handing it away, Cahoon returns. You explain what you saw but that you have no experience of injecting and Una was becoming uncomfortable. Cahoon appears to understand. '*Let me show you how I do it*', he says. Replacing the scope, he injects adrenaline into the bleeding point of the ulcer and the ooze stops. Withdrawing the scope, he tells you that he must go and help Halsted in theatre and he will see you later. Regarding the patient's proton pump inhibitor, the nurse wants to know if you want to:

I. Stop it ⋯⟩ **222**

II. Leave it as a once-daily dose ⋯⟩ **280**

III. Increase it to a twice-daily dose ⋯⟩ **241**

IV. Start a continuous infusion ⋯⟩ **226**

254 You calculate Marco's modified GCS and although only 24 hours into his symptoms, he scores two positive factors in his WBC and his pO_2.

⋯⟩ **213**

255 Susie heads away with her date for surgery. She returns 5 weeks later for her laparoscopic cholecystectomy. Cahoon is carrying out the surgery but becomes irate when he sees that nobody has advised her to lose weight, stop smoking or stop her contraceptive pill. **Deduct 1 point** and keep your head down.

⋯⟩ **279**

256 The lady and her daughter are grateful for your help. The next day the microbiology laboratory contacts you to say they have grown *Staph. aureus* in the ulcer sensitive to co-amoxyclav. You contact Mrs Nowak and start her on a 5-day course of antibiotics. Two weeks later Halsted receives a phone call from a local surgeon complaining that young nurses and doctors these days '*just wouldn't know a non-infected venous ulcer if it bit them. I'm sick of these kids throwing antibiotics around like sweets, do you guys train your doctors or what?*'. Halsted apologises on your behalf. Cringe and **deduct 1 point**.

⋯⟩ **183**

257 You wait but there is no sign of Cahoon returning and Una is becoming a little distressed as the scope irritates her duodenum. Do you want to:

I. Withdraw ⋯⟩ **253**

II. Inject ⋯⟩ **286**

258 Nicola becomes impatient and realising you don't know what you're doing, rings Cahoon who agrees to do an embolectomy under local anaesthetic. '*Not your finest hour, Simpson,*' he says. '*I'll look after this from here.*' Disappointed with yourself, you return to the slot. The next patient is the lady with right upper quadrant pain. Wearily you pull back the curtain.

⋯⟩ **247**

259 You administer oxygen through a face mask. Do you want to give nitrates?

I. Yes ⋯⟩ **248**

II. No ⋯⟩ **171**

260 With the help of her daughter, Norma explains that she has had a leg ulcer for nearly a month. It has been looked after by a local surgeon who recently changed her to a tight dressing, which has helped enormously. The ulcer has finally been reducing in size over the past 2 weeks. Today her normal nurse was away and she had a new nurse dress the wound. The new nurse was worried that the ulcer was infected and sent her to the emergency department. Mrs Nowak has no pain and generally feels well. She was never a smoker and is not a diabetic. Would you like to:

I. Order a blood count, ESR and CRP ⋯⟩ **300**

II. Order an x-ray ⋯⟩ **204**

III. Admit Norma for intravenous benzylpenicillin and flucloxacillin ⋯⟩ **318**

IV. Allow Norma home with a non-constricting dressing and a course of penicillin and flucloxacillin ⋯⟩ **180**

V. Replace the compression dressings that the nurse removed, reassure Norma and send her home to be followed up by her regular surgeon ⋯⟩ **232**

VI. Allow home, swab the ulcer and if positive prescribe a course of antibiotics appropriate to culture ⋯⟩ **256**

261 You are satisfied that she will be followed up in the clinic. In 4 weeks she will return to the clinic and will be reviewed by Cahoon, who pulls you out of your clinic room demanding to know why you've wasted his and the patient's time in not having her investigations complete before coming back to the clinic. '*It's just one mess-up after another with you, Simpson. Now*

I have to book her for an ultrasound and then get her back to schedule her for a cholecystectomy.' **Deduct 1 point**. However, right now, pleased with yourself, you return to the slot and pick up the chart of your next patient.

→ 279

262 You cover with ampicillin. **Add 1 point**.

→ 172

263 You decide against anticoagulating her. Two days later she sends off another clot, this time to her right leg, completely occluding her graft. The surgeon on call swears that if he ever finds out '*who decided not to give this woman anticoagulation, I'll string them up from the fifth floor*'. **Deduct 1 point**. You keep your head down for the next few days. You return to the slot – the next patient is the lady with right upper quadrant pain. Wearily, you pull back the curtain.

→ 247

264 Four weeks later, Cahoon leaves the clinic and starts roaring and shouting up and down the corridor looking for you, finally completely frustrated. **Deduct 1 point** and keep your head down.

→ 279

265 You decide to wait before performing an upper endoscopy. Una is taken to the ward for observation. Unfortunately, the ward is very busy and the staff do not appreciate the seriousness of Una's condition. You are reviewing another patient and about 1 hour later Una is found unresponsive and an arrest call is put out. You hear the arrest alarm and rush to the ward, finding the arrest team and Cahoon already there. Cahoon doesn't look up at you when you try to speak. Unfortunately, Una has been down for several minutes before being found and although the arrest team work hard for nearly 40 minutes, she dies. Cahoon curses and walks away, flinging his stethoscope across the nurses' desk. You try to follow but he turns and stops in the corridor. '*You left that girl bleeding on a ward, what the hell were you thinking, Simpson? Don't bother, you weren't thinking. I don't want you in this hospital, give me your bleep and get the hell out of here.*' You try to argue but he isn't listening. With your heart in your shoes, you hand over your bleep and leave Pilgrims for the cold night air. Maybe Pilgrims wasn't for you . . .

266 **Add 1 point**. Una is still mildly tachycardic at 104 and has had one more episode of haematemesis. She is alert and orientated. Do you want to perform an upper endoscopy now?

I. Yes ⋯⋗ **166**

II. No ⋯⋗ **265**

267 Just as you're about to give LMWH, Mia asks if that will cause a problem for any potential surgery later. Embarrassed, you tell her to go and get you a copy of Regina's x-rays from the radiology department, and when she leaves you decide to give UH instead. What will you do now?

I. Contact radiology to arrange an angiogram ⋯⋗ **251**

II. Contact Nicola to arrange an embolectomy ⋯⋗ **295**

268 Good. Although he does not make any urine initially, by the third litre he is putting out 25 ml per hour. Happy that he has had enough analgesia, what will you do next?

I. Give supplemental oxygen ⋯⋗ **186**

II. Order radiology ⋯⋗ **198**

III. Give antibiotics ⋯⋗ **235**

269 You contact radiology and organise a lower limb angiogram. Do you want Ruth to do a:

I. Formal angiogram ⋯⋗ **282**

II. CT angiogram ⋯⋗ **212**

270 Two hours later and the blood results come back. What will you do next?

I. Admit for intravenous benzylpenicillin and flucloxacillin ⋯⋗ **318**

II. Allow Norma home with a non-constricting dressing and a course of penicillin and flucloxacillin ⋯⋗ **180**

III. Allow Norma home, swab the ulcer and if positive prescribe a course of antibiotics appropriate to culture ⋯⋗ **256**

IV. Replace the compression dressings that the nurse removed, reassure Norma and send her home to be followed up by her regular surgeon ⋯⋗ **232**

271 The chest x-ray shows a small pleural effusion on the right side. However, as Marco is comfortable now and saturating normally, you decide to observe it. What do you want to do next?

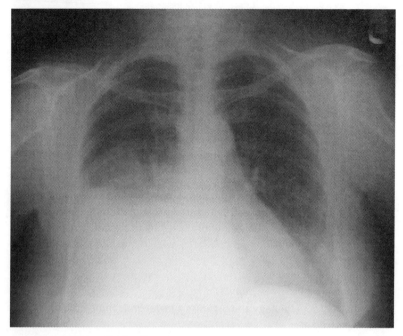

Chest x-ray of Marco Baldinelli.

I. Order an ultrasound ⋯⟩ 320

II. Order a CT abdomen ⋯⟩ 205

III. Start antibiotics and get a CT abdomen ⋯⟩ 203

272 You cross-match for two units and await Una's response to fluids. She vomits again, mostly coffee grounds but there are flecks of fresh blood also. Her pulse is 108 and BP is 100/70. Glad you cross-matched her for blood, do you want to now pass a Sengstaken–Blakemore tube?

I. Yes ⋯⟩ 214

II. No ⋯⟩ 187

273 Pulling back the curtain, you see Marco putting on his trousers and shirt. Una is behind him, pale and crying, pleading with him to stay. She looks up as you enter. '*Tell him to stay, doctor; please tell him to stay, he says he's going home.*' Will you:

I. Allow him to go ⋯⟩ 303

II. Try to reason with him ⋯⟩ 219

Section 2

274 Marco lies down flat on the trolley. His pulse is 112, BP 110/82, temp 37.1°C and O_2 saturations of 92%. His tongue is fissured and dry and he has involuntary guarding with localised rebound in his epigastric region. The rest of his abdomen is soft and non-tender. His blood results are available in the Investigations at the end of this section. What will you do next?

  I. Give him IV fluids ⋯⟩ **242**

  II. Give supplemental oxygen ⋯⟩ **290**

  III. Order radiology ⋯⟩ **198**

  IV. Take him to theatre immediately ⋯⟩ **313**

275 You give Norma a loading dose of clopidogrel.

  ⋯⟩ **305**

276 It's always worthwhile learning more by reading the charts first.

  ⋯⟩ **311**

277 You are happy with yourself that you are making a stand against smoking, and Susie leaves the department. In 8 months she will return to the ICU with gallstone pancreatitis. **Deduct 1 point.** You return to the slot and pick up the chart of your next patient.

  ⋯⟩ **279**

278 You pull back the curtain and he is leaning forward holding his epigastrium. Una Lordan, his girlfriend, is rubbing his back as you enter and they both look up. You introduce yourself and he grunts incomprehensibly at you. Una apologises and explains that he has been up all night with pain. You nod consolingly and tell them that you understand completely, while deep down you know this is going to be an awkward one. Do you:

  I. Take a history ⋯⟩ **201**

  II. Ask him to sit back, and examine him ⋯⟩ **245**

  III. Give analgesia ⋯⟩ **193**

279 The only chart left in the slot is that of the man with cellulitis. You call his name, but he does not answer. One of the receptionists thinks he might have gone outside for a cigarette. You take a quick look outside the entrance; the night air is chilly and as everybody seems pretty mobile, you reason that he'll turn up. You take the opportunity for a quick coffee upstairs. You climb the stairs wearily, the day beginning to take its toll, but you're nearly there. Calculate your scores from Section 2. (Please turn over).

280 You leave the proton pump inhibitor as a once-daily dose now that the bleeding has stopped and return to the slot. Tomorrow night, Winston is on call when Una rebleeds. As they wheel her to theatre, he takes great satisfaction telling Cahoon that the whole mess was avoidable but *'somebody'* hadn't read the latest literature on GI bleeding. Cahoon promises to look into it as Winston hands him Una's chart, open, of course, on the page with your note on it. **Deduct 1 point**.

⋯⊱ **299**

281 You begin to draw up the urokinase but Ubeki, the staff nurse, becomes concerned and tells you that it might be worthwhile contacting Cahoon or the cardiologist first. You contact Cahoon but he's tied up for 20 minutes. Do you wait to give the urokinase?

I. *Yes* ⋯⊱ **223**

II. *No* ⋯⊱ **202**

282 By the time it is performed and reported, nearly an hour has passed. Ruth tells you that there is a clear cut-off at the left distal superficial femoral artery, suggestive of an embolism. Do you want to:

I. *Start heparin* ⋯⊱ **211**

II. *Use thrombolysis* ⋯⊱ **233**

III. *Ring Nicola and organise and embolectomy* ⋯⊱ **295**

283 You advise her to stop her contraceptive pill before surgery and use alternative contraception, in order to reduce her risk of thrombosis. Happy to leave, you schedule her for surgery and let her go home.

⋯⊱ **279**

284 You arrive on the surgical ward and Regina is sitting up on the bed and appears quite comfortable. Her pulse is 74 and her BP is 138/78. She says she has no pain. Her pre-op ECG, tonight's ECG and her bloods can be found in the Investigations at the end of this section. She is only 12 days post op and Mia was afraid to give her aspirin. Do you:

I. *Give aspirin* ⋯⊱ **196**

II. *Not give aspirin* ⋯⊱ **239**

285 Susie comes back to the clinic 4 weeks later and is seen by Cahoon. He is a bit irritated that she was not simply booked for surgery rather than wasting his time at the clinic. **Deduct 1 point** and keep your head down.

⋯⟩ **279**

286 What would you like to inject with?

   I. Saline ⋯⟩ **173**

   II. Adrenaline ⋯⟩ **191**

287 This man is clearly your priority. You pull back the curtain and Marco Baldinelli is leaning forward holding his epigastrium. Una Lordan, his girlfriend, is rubbing his back as you enter and they both look up. You introduce yourself and he grunts incomprehensibly at you. Una apologises and explains that he has been up all night with pain. You nod consolingly and tell them that you understand completely, while deep down you know this is going to be an awkward one. Do you:

   I. Take a history ⋯⟩ **201**

   II. Ask him to sit back, and examine him ⋯⟩ **245**

   III. Give analgesia ⋯⟩ **193**

288 Susie is not impressed and scowls at you. You gently explain that she is carrying a little extra weight and that this will make the surgery more difficult and reduce her chances of a laparoscopic approach. **Add 1 point**. She seems to understand, but insists she must leave now for the remainder of her evening ball. What will you do next?

   I. Schedule surgery and allow her home, advising her to avoid fatty food ⋯⟩ **215**

   II. Tell her to stop smoking ⋯⟩ **207**

   III. Tell her to stop the oral contraceptive pill ⋯⟩ **224**

289 Her daughter says '*Of course*' and leaves for the waiting room. Norma puts down her book and smiles. Do you want to:

   I. Examine her ⋯⟩ **236**

   II. Take a history ⋯⟩ **250**

290 Yes, Marco is saturating poorly and certainly supplemental oxygen will help. **Give yourself 1 point**. You apply oxygen and his O_2 saturations slowly climb to 99%. What will you do next?

I. Give him IV fluids ⋯⟩ **238**

II. Order radiology ⋯⟩ **198**

III. Take him to theatre immediately ⋯⟩ **313**

291 You advise her to stop 3 weeks before surgery, as even this is a help. **Add 1 point**. Next do you:

I. Tell her to stop the contraceptive pill ⋯⟩ **283**

II. Schedule her for surgery and let her go home ⋯⟩ **319**

292 As you can see, Marco's CRP on admission is 134. You decide to check it again at 24 hours.

⋯⟩ **213**

293 She is at risk of further embolisation and so while she is being worked up and her condition controlled, she needs to be anticoagulated. **Add 1 point**. With her leg comfortable and pain free, you leave her in the hands of the cardiologist and plan to review her again later. Just as you're leaving the ward, you overhear one of the nurses talking to the lady's nephew. *'No, Mr Appleton, she can't make legal changes to her will now, as she is being assessed by the cardiologist and really she has not requested to see a legal representative. Yes, I appreciate that you are anxious to talk to her about it but you will really have to wait.'* You shake your head and return downstairs to the slot. The next patient is the lady with right upper quadrant pain. Tired now, you pull back the curtain.

⋯⟩ **247**

294 Susie tells you that *'I'll just die without my cigarettes, I've tried but it's impossible for me to go more than 4 weeks without them'*. Do you:

I. Refuse her surgery and send her away ⋯⟩ **277**

II. Tell her to give up 4 weeks before surgery ⋯⟩ **314**

III. Tell her not to worry about it ⋯⟩ **181**

295 It is likely that she has an embolus. Nicola tells you there is no way she is getting a general anaesthetic given that she has a probable MI. What will you do?

I. Argue for a GA ⋯⟩ **258**

II. Argue for a local anaesthetic ⋯⟩ **194**

III. Call Cahoon ⋯⟩ **199**

296 As she is not having an STEMI you decide not to thrombolyse her. **Add 1 point**. You get the heparin ready and are just calling the cardiologist with a view to further management when Regina complains that her left leg is painful. Examining her, you find the graft on the right is working normally, but her left leg is cold and painful to the level of the knee. She has no popliteal or distal pulses on the left side. Her movement and sensation are normal. What will you do next?

> I. Start heparin ⟶ **208**

> II. Contact radiology for a lower limb angiogram ⟶ **269**

> III. Contact Nicola and arrange an embolectomy in theatre ⟶ **295**

297 It's usually worthwhile reading the chart first in order to prioritise your patients, but clearly this man is your priority. You pull back the curtain and Marco Baldinelli is leaning forward holding his epigastrium. Una Lordan, his girlfriend, is rubbing his back as you enter and they both look up. You introduce yourself and he grunts incomprehensibly at you. Una apologises and explains that he has been up all night with pain. You nod consolingly and tell them that you understand completely, while deep down you know this is going to be an awkward one. Do you:

> I. Take a history ⟶ **201**

> II. Ask him to sit back, and examine him ⟶ **245**

> III. Give analgesia ⟶ **193**

298 Susie lies down, and you note from her chart that she has a BMI of about 31. Her vital signs are normal and her abdomen is soft and completely non-tender. Her bloods can be seen in the Investigations at the end of this section. She tells you that she has a evening dress ball tonight and really needs to leave to catch the end of it. What do you want to do next?

> I. Order radiology ⟶ **216**

> II. Allow her home but bring her back to the clinic ⟶ **322**

> III. Allow her home and not bring her back ⟶ **169**

299 You return to the slot but then Mia, your intern, rings you. *'Dr Simpson, I'm very sorry to be calling you but I have a patient I'm really worried about.'* She goes on to tell you about Regina Appleton, a 53 year old who is now 12 days post right femoral popliteal bypass for peripheral vascular disease and has been slow to mobilise. She is on a low prophylactic dose of LMWH. She was wheeled down to the front door of the hospital to have a cigarette when she developed chest pain, similar to the angina she suffers with activity, except this time she was at rest. Mia has given her oxygen,

Section 2

morphine and GTN, and the pain has settled. Her ECG is abnormal and Mia is worried that Regina may be having a myocardial infarction. You leave the emergency department to review Mrs Appleton.

⋯⟩ **284**

300 Two hours later and the blood results come back. Norma and her daughter are very anxious to leave, as they have been here more than 4 hours. What will you do next?

> I. *Order an x-ray* ⋯⟩ **197**

> II. *Admit Norma for intravenous benzylpenicillin and flucloxacillin* ⋯⟩ **318**

> III. *Allow Norma home with a non-constricting dressing and a course of penicillin and flucloxacillin* ⋯⟩ **180**

> IV. *Replace the compression dressings that the nurse removed and send Norma home to be followed up by her surgeon* ⋯⟩ **232**

> V. *Allow home, swab the ulcer and if positive prescribe a course of antibiotics appropriate to culture* ⋯⟩ **256**

301 OK, so you know that this isn't a good score. Scoring a negative figure shows that your basic knowledge could do with some brushing up, as well as adding to your experience in day-to-day decisions. However, it also shows that you're remarkably honest. This paragraph will be the one in the book that is least read, not because people don't score badly, they do, but because often people have trouble admitting it, if even to themselves, so well done. The only person that knows your score is you, and the only person who needs to make a difference is you. Make your mistakes with books like this, or websites or vignettes. In the past we 'practised' on patients, but that shouldn't be the way to learn now. Nicholas de Belleville, a French physician, once said, '*When you are called to a sick man, be sure you know what the matter is – if you do not know, nature can do a great deal better than you can guess*'. Chin up, you'll do just fine. Why not try repeating the section before you start on Section 3 and show yourself that while you have made your mistakes you've really improved because of them.

302 You give him 10 mg of morphine and cyclizine. Within a minute or two he has settled back into the trolley and looks considerably more comfortable. Will you:

> I. *Take a history* ⋯⟩ **221**

> II. *Examine him* ⋯⟩ **178**

303 Figuring that you've too much going on to worry about some guy who's drunk himself into a bad pancreatitis, you wish him good luck and head back out to the slot. Una looks on disbelievingly and runs out to Margaret. She rings Cahoon, who agrees to come in to try and reason with Marco. Feeling a little worried that Margaret has rung Cahoon, you slip back over to see what's happening. Just then Cahoon comes around the curtain, having scrubbed out of theatre. He has no idea who the patient is or what is going on, leaving you to hope that the ground opens up and swallows you, as you have some explaining to do. Just as Marco begins to shout again, Una suddenly vomits 500 ml of fresh blood onto the bed. Cahoon and Margaret quickly grab her, put her onto the next trolley and rush her to the resuscitation room, leaving a nurse and security guard to look after Marco. Just as Cahoon leaves, he glares at you: *'What have you been doing down here? Just get out, I'll look after it, you're a liability, Simpson'.* You try to reason amidst the chaos, but it's useless, he doesn't want to listen. You'll have to try explaining to Halsted in the morning that you've done nothing wrong.

304 Knowing that meropenem has the best pancreatic penetration, you draw it up and administer it intravenously. You are happy that he is comfortable and stable and that his urine output is adequate. Ruth calls you back and says that she has been studying the images and now sees a 2 cm cyst in the body of the pancreas. The whole picture certainly looks like that of an acute pancreatitis. Ruth asks if you want her to drain the cyst. Do you:

I. *Say yes* ⋯⋙ **244**

II. *Say no* ⋯⋙ **174**

III. *Ring Cahoon and ask his advice* ⋯⋙ **184**

305 It certainly seems that she has had an ischaemic event in her heart. Do you want to thrombolyse her?

I. *Yes* ⋯⋙ **281**

II. *No* ⋯⋙ **296**

306 Ruth is familiar with the literature supporting the use of thrombolysis in the setting of an embolus and she is willing to try. However, she laughs at you when you go to draw up the thrombolysis. *'What are you doing?'* she asks, grinning. When you try to explain, she suggests you ring Cahoon while she gets ready to administer localised thrombolysis.

⋯⋙ **167**

307 Una is alert but tachycardic at 120 with a BP of 90/70. Learning from your previous cases, you insert two large-bore IV cannulae and start fluid resuscitation. While you are inserting the catheter and taking bloods, Marco comes into the resus room behind you. *'She doesn't drink ordinarily,'* he explains, *'but I made her try and keep up with my drinking over the* *last 2 weeks.*' You ask if Una has any pain or other health problems. She tells you that she has no pain, has a cardiac murmur for which she is awaiting an echocardiogram, but is on no medications other than the oral contraceptive pill. She also tells you that her stool has been black and sticky for the past 3 days. Joy, the nurse, is about to send away the bloods. Do you want to:

I. Group and save ⇢ **246**

II. Cross-match ⇢ **272**

308 Marco's pulse rises and he becomes more lethargic. His urine output for the past hour is only 5 ml. Margaret becomes worried and rings Cahoon who tells her he can't leave theatre but to give 2 litres stat and '*get Simpson to reassess, I'll see him as soon as I can*'. By the time the second litre is finishing, Marco's urine output has risen to 20 ml per hour and you prescribe another litre of fluid. **Deduct 1 point**. What will you do next?

I. Order radiology ⇢ **198**

II. Give antibiotics ⇢ **235**

309 You hold off on the oxygen. Do you want to give nitrates?

I. Yes ⇢ **248**

II. No ⇢ **171**

310 You organise an ultrasound which confirms gallstones. At the next clinic you schedule surgery.

⇢ **279**

311 Clearly the other patient should have been your priority; **deduct 1 point**. The lady had one episode of right upper quadrant pain 5 hours ago lasting 2 hours. She is pain free now and her pulse is 72, BP 110/64, O_2 saturations 100% and temperature normal. The man has just returned from holiday with severe epigastric pain and vomiting. His pulse is 112, BP is 178/98, O_2 saturations 90% and temperature is normal. You walk over to the lady but she has left for a cigarette. So you go to see the man you should have prioritised.

⇢ **252**

312 You give morphine intravenously; **deduct 1 point**. Do you want to start a beta-blocker?

I. Yes ⇢ **200**

II. No ⇢ **177**

313 You ring your anaesthetist, Nicola Pablo, and book theatre for an emergency laparotomy. She becomes suspicious when you tell her that you're not sure what's going on but *'clearly this man needs a laparotomy'*. She reviews the patient herself and quite obviously sees that Marco is suffering a bad pancreatitis and needs fluid resuscitation and not surgery. She initiates resuscitation and phones Cahoon, telling him that his new doc is a loose cannon. Horrified, Cahoon comes in and tells you to *'get the hell out of this department; I'll look after the patients tonight'*. You try to explain but he's fuming: *'Tell it to Halsted in the morning'*. You pick up your stuff and can't help feeling that you've seen your last patient in Pilgrims.

314 You advise her to stop 4 weeks before surgery, as even this is a help. **Add 1 point**. You schedule her surgery and let her go home.

⋯⟩ **279**

315 Four weeks later at the clinic, Cahoon leaves his room and starts roaring and shouting up and down the corridor looking for you, finally completely frustrated. **Deduct 1 point** and keep your head down.

⋯⟩ **279**

316 You give a bolus of heparin and start an infusion. **Add 1 point**. What will you do now?

   I. Contact radiology to arrange an angiogram ⋯⟩ **251**

   II. Contact Nicola to arrange an embolectomy ⋯⟩ **295**

317 Susie tells you that *'I'll just die without my cigarettes, I've tried but it's impossible for me to go more than a few weeks without them'*. Do you:

   I. Refuse her surgery and send her away ⋯⟩ **277**

   II. Tell her to give up 4 weeks before surgery ⋯⟩ **314**

   III. Tell her not to worry about it ⋯⟩ **181**

318 Samuel Norman, the bed co-ordinator, asks why this patient needed to come in, as they are desperately short of beds tonight. You tell him the patient needs IV antibiotics and he must find her a bed. The following morning the lady is no longer in the hospital. As Halsted does a ward round, Cahoon whispers that he saved both of you the embarrassment of having to explain what a patient with a chronic non-infected ulcer was doing occupying an emergency bed. **Deduct 1 point**.

⋯⟩ **183**

319 Susie heads away with her date for surgery. She returns 5 weeks later for her laparoscopic cholecystectomy. Cahoon is carrying out the surgery but becomes irate when he sees that nobody has advised her to stop her contraceptive pill. **Deduct 1 point** and keep your head down.

⋯⟩ **279**

320 There are no gallstones in the gallbladder, but it is difficult to see the pancreas as it is obscured by gas-filled loops of bowel. What would you like to do next?

   I. Order a CT abdomen ⋯⟩ **205**

   II. Start antibiotics and order a CT abdomen ⋯⟩ **203**

321 You are just calling the cardiologist with a view to further management and are about to start heparin, when Regina complains that her left leg is painful. Examining her, you find the graft on the right is working normally, but her left leg is cold and painful to the level of the knee. She has no popliteal or distal pulses on the left side. Her movement and sensation are normal. What will you do next?

   I. Start heparin ⋯⟩ **208**

   II. Contact radiology for a lower limb angiogram ⋯⟩ **269**

   III. Contact Nicola and arrange theatre ⋯⟩ **295**

322 What would you like to request, so that the result is available when she returns to clinic?

   I. PFA ⋯⟩ **264**

   II. Ultrasound abdomen ⋯⟩ **310**

   III. CT abdomen ⋯⟩ **315**

323 Ruth becomes impatient. *'Listen, I've got this guy on the table now and it's late. If you want me to drain it I'll do it now, otherwise I'm going home.'* What do you want to do?

   I. Drain ⋯⟩ **244**

   II. Don't drain ⋯⟩ **174**

324 You wheel Una into the resuscitation room, your own pulse quickening.

⋯⟩ **307**

325 Ruth is familiar with the literature supporting the use of thrombolysis in the setting of an embolus and she is willing to try.

⋯⟩ **167**

326 You give the enteric-coated aspirin; **deduct 1 point**. Do you want to administer oxygen?

I. Yes ⋯⟩ **259**

II. No ⋯⟩ **309**

327 You decide to hold off on the antibiotics; **deduct 1 point**.

⋯⟩ **172**

PERSPECTIVES

Case perspectives: Norma Nowak

THERAPEUTIC PERSPECTIVES

1 Rationalising investigations: bloods/x-ray

- It has been estimated that between 25%[1] and 42%[2] of laboratory tests ordered in the emergency department are inappropriate.
- A Canadian-based report has shown that between the 1970s and 1990s, the ordering of tests has increased by 130%.[3]
- The cause of this increase has been multifactorial and includes:
  - fear of criticism by seniors[4]
  - the concept of 'routine' diagnostic testing[5]
  - excessive repeat testing[6]
  - the entertainment of obscure diagnoses by junior staff[4]
  - irrelevant test results stimulating further inappropriate follow-on tests.[7]
- Where clinical suspicion exists, ESR, CRP and WBC can be useful to diagnose a wound infection. Similarly plain x-rays can be helpful when osteomyelitis is suspected.[8]

NORMA AND INVESTIGATIONS

Neither the history nor the examination suggests that the ulcer is infected or that there is underlying osteomyelitis. If you ordered the inflammatory blood tests and the x-ray, Norma and her daughter grew weary and left the department. If this happened you were deducted 1 point.

2 Swabs and antibiotics for non-infected wounds

- Warmth, erythema and discharge are signs of active infection. Chronic ulcers* may not always display all these signs, but increased pain, malodour, increased friability, extension or breakdown of the wound surface should raise the possibility of underlying infection or bone involvement.[9,10]
- All wounds become contaminated, regardless of prevention strategies.[11]
- Swabs should be used as an adjunct rather than as the basis for a diagnosis of infection of a chronic ulcer.[8]
- The use of topical or systemic antibiotics is not recommended to prevent colonisation* of chronic ulcers.[8,12]

*please refer to the Definitions at the end of this Case perspective.

- Currently there is no evidence to support the use of systemic antibiotics to promote the healing of chronic venous ulcers.[13] While a recent Cochrane* review has acknowledged that there is a lack of reliable evidence in the area, because of the danger presented by bacterial resistance, systemic antibiotics should be given only for cases of defined infection.[13]

NORMA AND SWABS AND ANTIBIOTICS

As mentioned previously, there is no evidence that this wound is infected, and the fact that it has shown dramatic improvement over the past 2 weeks supports this. Swabbing this wound is likely to give you only the organisms which inevitably are colonising it. Furthermore, giving antibiotics, either by admitting Norma or allowing her home on oral antibiotics, is both a waste of resources and bad practice. If you decided to admit Norma, you would have been chastised by Cahoon the following morning and deducted a point. Similarly, if you allowed Norma home on oral antibiotics, regardless of swab results, her surgeon would have written complaining that '*Young nurses and doctors these days just wouldn't know a non-infected venous ulcer if it bit them*'. If this happened you were also deducted 1 point.

3 Compression for venous ulcers

- The prevalence of active leg ulceration in the developed world has been estimated at approximately 1.5/1000.[14,15]
- The exact aetiology remains unclear but venous ulceration appears to be related to increased hydrostatic pressure* in the veins of the leg. Reversing this and aiding venous return is the principle of compression therapy.[16]
- Graduated* elastic compression* increases femoral vein blood flow[17] and decreases venous pressure distally.[18]
- Venous ulcers heal more rapidly with compression than without.[16]
- Multi-component* bandaging/stockings are more effective than single component, and multi-component bandaging/stockings containing elastic elements are more effective than those that are inelastic.[16]
- Compression dressings may reduce blood supply to distal tissue so before initiating compression therapy, patients should be screened for arterial disease, including the use of the Ankle Brachial Index (ABI).[19]
- Patients with ABI* greater than 0.85 can usually be safely treated with compression.[20] However, it should be remembered that patients with calcified vessels can have a falsely elevated ABI.
- Patients with ABI between 0.5 and 0.7 may only be eligible for *modified* compression treatment.[21]

NORMA AND COMPRESSION

It is clear from a properly taken history that Norma's ulcer is improving, with the 'tight dressings' initiated by Norma's surgeon. If you elected to remove or replace them, you were deducted points and her surgeon would have written a letter of complaint. Maintaining the compression, which was well tolerated, was the right course of action, gaining you the most marks.

COMMUNICATION PERSPECTIVES

Public health nurse's perspective

• The public health nurse has never seen this ulcer before.
• She has not practised for over 7 months and is covering for a colleague who is away.
• She is anxious not to make any mistakes while covering, as she is looking for a permanent job.
• She has a low threshold for referring in any patient she is unsure about.

SIMPSON AND THE PUBLIC HEALTH NURSE

It is irritating that you have been made to deal with a patient unnecessarily, particularly as you are busy with many other, more serious patients. One of the first impulses one feels is to pick up the phone and tell this to the public health nurse. While this might allow you to vent your frustration, it is worth stopping for a moment before dialling the number. Regardless of your call, you must deal with the situation as it is. In terms of the clinical problems you will face, it is an easy one. Embarrassing or shouting at a colleague will not help achieve that particular task, it will only consume another few precious minutes in what is a long night, possibly breaking your concentration for the next patient you see. Often what you deem as an inappropriate referral may in fact be a cry for help from a colleague who, for whatever reason, finds themselves out of their depth. In such a case, the most important priority is ensuring that the patient is safe. Afterwards, if you managed to resist the temptation to shout at your colleague, perhaps a more informal call to let them know how the patient got on, and to suggest a possible way in which they could manage the patient next time, might work better.

Surgeon's perspective

• The surgeon has been treating Norma for the past 2 weeks.
• He has made a diagnosis and initiated a treatment plan.
• The treatment plan involves compression therapy and time.

- He has made plans to review her after an interval long enough so that he can see results.
- By changing his treatment plan, he will not see the results he hopes for.

SIMPSON AND THE SURGEON

Looking at the case from the surgeon's perspective, he has diagnosed and treated Norma and is waiting to see the results of his treatment plan. Unlike the treatment of many medical conditions, the resolution of chronic ulcers can take a considerable amount of time and so he has probably left Norma for a decent interval before seeing her again. If you change his diagnosis and treatment plan, it will set back her recovery, causing him to have to start again. For this reason, it is not surprising that he is upset. While some may have elected to speak to you directly, he has decided to complain to Halsted. Unfortunately, this is sometimes the case, as many doctors feel it necessary to talk from 'peer to peer'. Ultimately the end result is probably the same as you are unlikely to make the same mistake twice.

Halsted's perspective

- The chief is in charge of the unit.
- A poor performance from the unit is a poor reflection on him.
- An external complaint is embarrassing, as is having to apologise for somebody else.

SIMPSON AND HALSTED

If your decisions resulted in the surgeon writing to the chief, you have managed to make your boss look bad. While some may not be too concerned at this, it is naive to think that this will not affect how successful this job is going to be for you. While our job as doctors is not to make others 'look good', certainly making your boss look bad is not going to help.

Perspective of Norma and her daughter

- Norma and her daughter have been dealing with the ulcer for a month now.
- The ulcer has been dressed daily and they have witnessed the improvement over the past 2 weeks.
- They are a little bemused at having to attend the emergency department. However, they take the advice of the public health nurse and seek attention.
- Waiting for a series of laboratory and radiological tests causes them to become impatient and they leave.

SIMPSON, NORMA AND HER DAUGHTER

Although you must preserve the patient's right of privacy, in this case it is clear that Norma wanted her daughter to stay. If you allowed this, you were rewarded with more information and the key point that neither Norma nor her daughter is worried about the ulcer. Allowing Norma to decide who she wants at the consultation is probably the best approach. If you delayed them with a series of tests, they became tired and left. This can be understood if you consider that they were only attending reluctantly in the first place.

What happened to Norma?

Norma continued to be managed with graded compression by her surgeon. Overall, her treatment required several months of compression but it was possible to heal her ulcer eventually and she is currently wearing compression stockings as prophylaxis.

DEFINITIONS

Chronic ulcer – a long-standing lesion where the surface tissue has been eroded and fails to heal normally.

Colonisation – the population of the surface of an area by a particular organism.

Compression – to squeeze or press together.

Cochrane – the Cochrane Collaboration is a non-profit group involving experts working together to analyse healthcare research.

Graduated – divided into degrees.

Hydrostatic pressure – the pressure exerted by a fluid at equilibrium at a given point.

Multi-component – having several elements.

ABI (Ankle Brachial Index) – the measure of the reduced blood pressure in the lower limbs.

REFERENCE LIST

1. Smellie WS, Murphy MJ, Galloway PJ, Hinnie J, McIlroy J, Dryburgh FJ. Audit of an emergency biochemistry service. J Clin Pathol 1995;48(12):1126–1129.
2. Perraro F, Rossi P, Liva C, et al. Inappropriate emergency test ordering in a general hospital: preliminary reports. Qual Assur Health Care 1992;4(1):77–81.
3. Ontario Ministry of Health. *Salient Features of the Laboratory Industry in Ontario 1992–1993.* Toronto: Ontario Ministry of Health, 1995.
4. Hardison JE. To be complete. N Engl J Med 1979;300(21):1225.
5. Routine diagnostic testing. Lancet 1989;2(8673):1190–1191.

6. Fraser CG. *Interpretation of Clinical Chemical Laboratory Data*. Oxford: Blackwell Scientific, 1986.

7. World Health Organization Working Group. *Assessment of Benefits and Costs of Clinical Laboratory Testing*. Geneva: World Health Organization, 1984.

8. Bergstrom N, Bennett M, Carlson C. *Treatment of Pressure Ulcers*. Clinical Practice Guideline No. 15. Publication No. 95-0652. Rockville, MD: US Department of Health and Human Services, Public Health Service, Agency for Health Care Policy and Research, 1994.

9. Gardner SE, Frantz RA, Doebbeling BN. The validity of the clinical signs and symptoms used to identify localized chronic wound infection. Wound Repair Regen 2001;9(3):178–186.

10. Gardner SE, Frantz RA, Troia C, et al. A tool to assess clinical signs and symptoms of localized infection in chronic wounds: development and reliability. Ostomy Wound Manage 2001;47(1):40–47.

11. Frank C, Bayoumi I, Westendorp C. Approach to infected skin ulcers. Can Fam Physician 2005;51:1352–1359.

12. O'Meara SM, Cullum NA, Majid M, Sheldon TA. Systematic review of antimicrobial agents used for chronic wounds. Br J Surg 2001;88(1):4–21.

13. O'Meara S, Al-Kurdi D, Ovington LG. Antibiotics and antiseptics for venous leg ulcers. Cochrane Database Syst Rev 2008;1:CD003557.

14. Lees TA, Lambert D. Prevalence of lower limb ulceration in an urban health district. Br J Surg 1992;79(10):1032–1034.

15. Baker SR, Stacey MC, Jopp-McKay AG, Hoskin SE, Thompson PJ. Epidemiology of chronic venous ulcers. Br J Surg 1991;78(7):864–867.

16. O'Meara S, Cullum NA, Nelson EA. Compression for venous leg ulcers. Cochrane Database Syst Rev 2009;1:CD000265.

17. Sigel B, Edelstein AL, Felix WR Jr, Memhardt CR. Compression of the deep venous system of the lower leg during inactive recumbency. Arch Surg 1973;106(1):38–43.

18. Somerville JJ, Brow GO, Byrne PJ, Quill RD, Fegan WG. The effect of elastic stockings on superficial venous pressures in patients with venous insufficiency. Br J Surg 1974;61(12):979–981.

19. Royal College of Nursing. *Clinical Practice Guideline: The Nursing Management of Patients with Venous Leg Ulcers*. London: Royal College of Nursing, 2006.

20. Ghauri AS, Nyamekye I, Grabs AJ, Farndon JR, Poskitt KR. The diagnosis and management of mixed arterial/venous leg ulcers in community-based clinics. Eur J Vasc Endovasc Surg 1998;16(4):350–355.

21. Moffatt C. *Compression Therapy in Practice*. Wounds Publishing UK, 2007. www.woundsuk.co.uk/journal.shtml

Case perspectives: Marco Baldinelli

THERAPEUTIC PERSPECTIVES

1 Prioritising your patients

- Marco has a tachycardia and low O_2 saturations.
- The lady has no symptoms and normal vital signs.

MARCO AND PRIORITISING

Marco clearly needs your attention sooner than the lady. If you choose to see her first you were deducted marks.

2 Analgesia for pancreatitis

- Patients with acute pancreatitis should have analgesia as a priority.
- Traditionally there has been a belief that giving morphine can make pain worse by causing spasm of the sphincter of Oddi,* thus raising biliary pressure, an effect which is not entirely reversed by naloxone.[1]
- It has been proposed that pethidine (merperidine) does not cause similar spasm[2] and so should be preferentially used in pancreatitis.[3]
- It has further been proposed that in patients who still have a gallbladder, the organ can accommodate the bile produced by the liver during times of spasm, thus avoiding rises in biliary pressure. Patients who have had a cholecystectomy do not have this capacity and thus experience a rise in biliary pressure during spasm.[4]
- More recently, some authors have argued that as all opioid-based drugs result in some increase in sphincter of Oddi pressure, morphine may actually be preferable as it provides longer acting relief from pain with less chance of seizures.[5]

MARCO AND ANALGESIA

Marco needs strong analgesia. The prescribing of this earned you 1 point. The difficulty with the debate surrounding pethidine versus morphine is the real lack of outcome-based studies comparing these two drugs in patients with acute pancreatitis. For us, there is still not enough clinical evidence to convince us that pethidine is superior to morphine in acute pancreatitis. For this reason you were awarded equal marks for relieving Marco's pain, regardless of how you achieved this.

*please refer to the Definitions at the end of this Case perspective.

3 Initial management

- Increased endothelial permeability results in oedema and this, accompanied by large third space fluid loss and hypovolaemia, increases the risk of further complications such as renal failure.[6]
- The importance of rapidly restoring and maintaining intravascular fluid volumes in acute pancreatitis has previously been clearly demonstrated.[7,8]
- While fluid resuscitation is essential, there are currently no convincing guidelines as to exactly what type of fluid or what volume of fluid is required.[9,10]

MARCO AND FLUIDS

Marco is clearly dehydrated and requires aggressive volume resuscitation. Biochemically, his urea is raised along with his lactate on ABG. Giving 500 ml over 1 hour fails to produce an adequate urine output and is insufficient. Giving 2 litres stat followed by 1 litre over 2 hours and then titrating the volume to his urine output gives you a far better result. This approach resulted in points being awarded. However, it should be remembered that patients with pancreatitis can often require as aggressive or more aggressive regimens than this, and should be monitored closely.

4 Effusion in pancreatitis

- Pleural complications are clinically or radiologically evident in 33% of patients with acute pancreatitis.[11] These include atelectasis, effusions, infiltrate, oedema and respiratory distress syndrome.
- A pleural effusion in acute pancreatitis is a poor prognostic sign.[12]
- The majority of pleural effusions (68%) are left-sided, 22% are bilateral and 10% are right-sided only. Two of the main causes are thought to be a transdiaphragmatic lymphatic blockage and a pancreaticopleural fistula.[13]
- The management of pleural effusions is initially conservative. However, some may require drainage. The majority of effusions will settle with the resolution of intra-abdominal inflammation.

MARCO AND EFFUSION

Marco has a reactive pleural effusion. Although he has decreased O_2 saturations initially, these rise with supplemental oxygen, earning you 1 point. An initially conservative approach to Marco's effusion would be appropriate.

5 Imaging in pancreatitis

- In cases where the presentation and blood results are characteristic of pancreatitis, there is probably no need for initial CT confirmation.[14] However, initial CT is useful in distinguishing pancreatitis from other alternative pathologies such as perforation or ischaemia.
- Ultrasound is important to establish the presence or absence of gallstones. However, in the actual assessment of the pancreas it is limited in its use, as often the pancreas is obscured by loops of gas-filled bowel and it is difficult to assess extraperitoneal extension of inflammation and fluid.[15]
- MRI has a similar ability to CT but is better for imaging the ductal system. However, it is often difficult to get in the acute setting and the image acquisition time is longer.
- It is well known that renal impairment may be worsened by intravenous contrast for CT. However, it is emerging that gadolinium, the contrast used in MRI scanning, may also be linked to nephrogenic systemic fibrosis.[16]
- Pancreatic necrosis usually occurs in the first 24–48 hours and imaging plays an important role in monitoring for its presence.[17]
- Some institutions use CT-based grading systems to determine prognosis.[18]

MARCO AND IMAGING

In Marco's case an ultrasound failed to demonstrate the pancreas adequately. However, having studied the films, your radiologist is happy that she can see a cyst. The CT was more definitive. As either of these imaging modalities would be appropriate where the diagnosis is almost certain, you were awarded equal marks for both options.

6 Pseudocyst

- A pancreatic pseudocyst is a localised fluid collection rich in amylase and enzymes, surrounded by a wall of fibrous tissue not lined by epithelium.[19]
- Pseudocysts are connected with the pancreatic ductal system, either directly or indirectly, and are caused by duct disruption resulting from duct obstruction from calculi, inflammation, necrosis or stenosis.[20]
- A pseudocyst takes 4–6 weeks to mature, whereas in contrast an acute fluid collection arises in the setting of acute pancreatitis and is characterised by a collection of non-enzymatic fluid that is the result of the acute inflammatory response, but not a complication of a disrupted pancreatic duct. An acute fluid collection invariably resolves spontaneously as the inflammatory process wanes.[21]
- Pseudocysts are less common after acute than chronic pancreatitis, but are more common in alcohol-induced pancreatitis.[20]

Section 2

- Some studies, including that by Vitas & Sarr, have shown that larger cysts are more likely to cause complications.[22]
- Most pseudocysts resolve spontaneously with supportive medical care only.[23]
- However, some large cysts do respond to conservative management (as did seven patients with cysts of 10 cm or more in the aforementioned study by Vitas & Sarr[22]) and so size is not an absolute indication for intervention.[24]
- The main reason for intervention is either symptoms or complications (infection, bleeding, biliary or gastric outlet obstruction).[20]
- Radiological drainage of the pseudocyst under ultrasound or CT guidance is usually performed by placing a drain into the cyst and allowing continuous drainage until the flow stops. Using this method, up to 50% of cysts can be resolved but it does increase the risk of infection.[20]
- The other options for draining pseudocysts are surgical or endoscopic drainage. Endoscopic drainage allows the cyst to drain internally into the duodenum or stomach. This technique is less invasive than surgery and some studies have reported a 90% success rate in dealing with pseudocysts from chronic pancreatitis.[25]

MARCO AND PSEUDOCYST

Marco's CT scan has demonstrated a small acute pseudocyst. This probably really represents an acute fluid collection. It is clear from this that your radiologist has limited experience in dealing with acute pancreatitis. A conservative approach involving re-imaging at a later time is indicated. Draining the cyst in the manner described, by simply aspirating, may introduce infection and is unlikely to be successful as the cyst may simply fill again. If you decided to aspirate or you were bullied into allowing the radiologist to aspirate, you were deducted points.

7 Antibiotics

- A very controversial subject and it is based on the assumption that preventing necrotic pancreatic tissue from becoming infected would improve outcome.
- Infection of pancreatic necrosis occurs in 40–70% of patients in the second or third week and is the leading cause of mortality and morbidity in pancreatitis.[26]
- Some studies have shown an advantage of prophylactic antibiotics[27,28] while others have failed to reproduce this.[29]
- Currently accepted practice is that when infection is suspected, and a fine needle aspiration has been performed, meropenem or imipenem is

commenced.[30] Treatment is continued for 14 days or stopped if infection is not confirmed.[26]

- Debridement or drainage may need to be performed for collections, necrotic material or abscesses, but only when tissues are infected.[31]
- When necrosis is sterile, mortality is low and patients can be managed conservatively.[26]
- Necrosis is monitored closely with repeated imaging and aspiration if patients show signs of deterioration.[31,32]

MARCO AND ANTIBIOTICS

While the CT result indicates a 20% reduction in the perfusion of the pancreas, there is no proof that Marco has infection at this very early stage of his pancreatitis. Currently, in our practice we apply the principles described above, and in this instance would not have administered antibiotics. However, we recognise that the evidence is far from clear and is often conflicting, and while we, like most units, advocate this approach, you were not deducted marks for deviating from this.

8 Self-discharge

- It has been estimated that 1–2% of medical admissions result in a discharge against medical advice.[33]
- Predictors include younger age, no health insurance, males, and current or a history of substance or alcohol abuse.[33]
- One recent UK study concluded that the standard self-discharge forms used in many UK emergency departments have no useful clinical role, and have little legal weight in protecting the hospital against litigation, often ignoring the patient's 'capacity' to consent.[34]
- When faced with a difficult case where a patient wants to self-discharge against medical advice, the doctors involved should try to present the information in a manner that enhances comprehension.[35]
- In certain circumstances the intervention of psychiatric services may help clarify the issue of capacity and sometimes can help successfully mediate between the patient and the team.[36]

MARCO AND SELF-DISCHARGE

Marco is clearly unwell. Although, with capacity, ultimately his decision to decline treatment is his own, you have an obligation to ensure that he understands the consequences fully. If you decided to let him go without attempting this, you were deducted points.

COMMUNICATION PERSPECTIVES

Una's perspective

- Clearly, from what subsequently happens, Una is not feeling well either.
- Her relationship with Marco does not allow her to express this. This must be a concern.
- The first indication that we get from Una that she is unwell is when she collapses with haematemesis.
- Una has been with Marco for over a year now. Although you are not told, there have been two occasions on which Marco has hit Una.

SIMPSON AND UNA

You are unaware of the dynamics between Una and Marco, and in the initial stages of treatment it is not as important as stabilising, diagnosing and treating your patient, who is, in this instance, Marco. However, as the case unfolds and particularly when it comes to eventually discharging our patients, we have a responsibility to know that we are discharging them to a safe environment. If we are in doubt regarding this, then we have a responsibility to improve it, in whatever way we can. When it is an adult involved, this will start with talking to the individual and bringing in whatever social and professional support you think may help.

Nurse's perspective

- Marco is dehydrated.
- If you gave just 500 ml as a stat dose, your prescription of intravenous fluids is inadequate.
- The initial priority for a patient with pancreatitis is rehydration.

SIMPSON AND MARGARET

Margaret is rightly concerned that Marco is being inadequately rehydrated. Her priority is the patient and so she must act on these concerns. She has two choices: either she voices her concerns to you or she goes above your head. In this instance she goes above your head. This is obviously not the approach you would prefer. There are most likely two explanations: either she does not trust you or alternatively her practice has shown her that it is quicker to go to the top. How you deal with this is going to define your relationship with this particular nurse for the rest of your rotation. Your choices are as follows.

1. Ignore it and continue to work in the hope of earning the confidence of your nursing colleagues. **This is the passive approach, but not to say the**

incorrect one. It will take longer to achieve change but does avoid direct and potentially unpleasant confrontation.

2. Confront Margaret with the intention of protesting that she went above your head. **This approach is fraught with potential difficulties. In our experience it often makes the situation worse, and is likely to result in Margaret becoming defensive and ultimately cause an unpleasant and public argument.**

3. Speak to Margaret informally, explaining that you're happy with any advice she can offer while you're finding your feet and that you're anxious to make a good impression. Explain that if she is worried about any of your decisions she should mention it to you first and if there's still a disagreement, you can both seek the advice of senior colleague. **This may represent a toned-down version of the second option, where you can potentially see quick results but yet more than likely avoid a direct argument. In our experience this approach followed by option 1 often yields the best results.**

What happened to Marco?

Marco was a very difficult patient to manage. He went on to have a prolonged stay in hospital complicated by ventilation for ARDS and eventually a necrosectomy for infected necrotic pancreatic tissue. As a consequence, when he was eventually discharged 7 weeks after his initial admission, he developed chronic pain and diabetes. He is still a regular visitor to the emergency department with complaints of pain and erratic sugars. His last admission was for diabetic ketoacidosis and he is poorly compliant with his insulin. As a result of his chronic pancreatitis, he is regularly assessed by the dietetics team and is on supplemental oral enzymes. However, he remains markedly underweight, having lost 30 kg since admission, and now has a BMI of just 17. He has been unable to work and is on disability benefits and overall his prognosis is poor, particularly because of his inability to comply with treatment. He remains a frustrating case.

DEFINITIONS

Sphincter of Oddi – the sphincter/muscle between the common bile duct and the pancreatic duct.

REFERENCE LIST

1. Helm JF, Venu RP, Geenen JE, et al. Effects of morphine on the human sphincter of Oddi. Gut 1988;29(10):1402–1407.
2. Wu SD, Zhang ZH, Jin JZ, et al. Effects of narcotic analgesic drugs on human Oddi's sphincter motility. World J Gastroenterol 2004;10(19):2901–2904.

3. Baker JE, Hearse DJ. Differing potencies and dose-response characteristics in the ability of slow-calcium-channel blockers to reduce enzyme leakage in the calcium paradox. Adv Myocardiol 1985;6:637–646.

4. Coelho JC, Senninger N, Runkel N, Herfarth C, Messmer K. Effect of analgesic drugs on the electromyographic activity of the gastrointestinal tract and sphincter of Oddi and on biliary pressure. Ann Surg 1986;204(1):53–58.

5. Thompson DR. Narcotic analgesic effects on the sphincter of Oddi: a review of the data and therapeutic implications in treating pancreatitis. Am J Gastroenterol 2001;96(4):1266–1272.

6. Tenner S. Initial management of acute pancreatitis: critical issues during the first 72 hours. Am J Gastroenterol 2004;99(12):2489–2494.

7. Klar E, Herfarth C, Messmer K. Therapeutic effect of isovolemic hemodilution with dextran 60 on the impairment of pancreatic microcirculation in acute biliary pancreatitis. Ann Surg 1990;211(3):346–353.

8. Wilmer A. ICU management of severe acute pancreatitis. Eur J Intern Med 2004;15(5):274–280.

9. Boldt J. Volume therapy in the intensive care patient – we are still confused, but . . . Intens Care Med 2000;26(9):1181–1192.

10. Eckerwall G, Olin H, Andersson B, Andersson R. Fluid resuscitation and nutritional support during severe acute pancreatitis in the past: what have we learned and how can we do better? Clin Nutr 2006;25(3):497–504.

11. Interiano B, Stuard ID, Hyde RW. Acute respiratory distress syndrome in pancreatitis. Ann Intern Med 1972;77(6):923–926.

12. Heller SJ, Noordhoek E, Tenner SM, et al. Pleural effusion as a predictor of severity in acute pancreatitis. Pancreas 1997;15(3):222–225.

13. Browne GW, Pitchumoni CS. Pathophysiology of pulmonary complications of acute pancreatitis. World J Gastroenterol 2006;12(44):7087–7096.

14. Banks PA, Freeman ML. Practice guidelines in acute pancreatitis. Am J Gastroenterol 2006;101(10):2379–2400.

15. Jeffrey RB Jr, Laing FC, Wing VW. Extrapancreatic spread of acute pancreatitis: new observations with real-time US. Radiology 1986;159(3):707–711.

16. Sadowski EA, Bennett LK, Chan MR, et al. Nephrogenic systemic fibrosis: risk factors and incidence estimation. Radiology 2007;243(1):148–157.

17. Kim DH, Pickhardt PJ. Radiologic assessment of acute and chronic pancreatitis. Surg Clin North Am 2007;87(6):1341–58, viii.

18. Balthazar EJ, Robinson DL, Megibow AJ, Ranson JH. Acute pancreatitis: value of CT in establishing prognosis. Radiology 1990;174(2):331–336.

19. Bradley EL III. A clinically based classification system for acute pancreatitis. Summary of the International Symposium on Acute Pancreatitis, Atlanta, GA, September 11 through 13, 1992. Arch Surg 1993;128(5):586–590.

20. Habashi S, Draganov PV. Pancreatic pseudocyst. World J Gastroenterol 2009;15(1):38–47.

21. Behrns KE, Ben-David K. Surgical therapy of pancreatic pseudocysts. J Gastrointest Surg 2008;12(12):2231–2239.

22. Vitas GJ, Sarr MG. Selected management of pancreatic pseudocysts: operative versus expectant management. Surgery 1992;111(2):123–130.

23. Yeo CJ, Bastidas JA, Lynch-Nyhan A, Fishman EK, Zinner MJ, Cameron JL. The natural history of pancreatic pseudocysts documented by computed tomography. Surg Gynecol Obstet 1990;170(5):411–417.

24. Cheruvu CV, Clarke MG, Prentice M, Eyre-Brook IA. Conservative treatment as an option in the management of pancreatic pseudocyst. Ann R Coll Surg Engl 2003;85(5):313–316.

25. Norton ID, Clain JE, Wiersema MJ, DiMagno EP, Petersen BT, Gostout CJ. Utility of endoscopic ultrasonography in endoscopic drainage of pancreatic pseudocysts in selected patients. Mayo Clin Proc 2001;76(8):794–798.

26. Frossard JL, Steer ML, Pastor CM. Acute pancreatitis. Lancet 2008;371(9607):143–152.

27. Sainio V, Kemppainen E, Puolakkainen P, et al. Early antibiotic treatment in acute necrotising pancreatitis. Lancet 1995;346(8976):663–667.

28. Delcenserie R, Yzet T, Ducroix JP. Prophylactic antibiotics in treatment of severe acute alcoholic pancreatitis. Pancreas 1996;13(2):198–201.

29. Isenmann R, Runzi M, Kron M, et al. Prophylactic antibiotic treatment in patients with predicted severe acute pancreatitis: a placebo-controlled, double-blind trial. Gastroenterology 2004;126(4):997–1004.

30. Heinrich S, Schafer M, Rousson V, Clavien PA. Evidence-based treatment of acute pancreatitis: a look at established paradigms. Ann Surg 2006;243(2):154–168.

31. Werner J, Feuerbach S, Uhl W, Buchler MW. Management of acute pancreatitis: from surgery to interventional intensive care. Gut 2005;54(3):426–436.

32. Uhl W, Warshaw A, Imrie C, et al. IAP guidelines for the surgical management of acute pancreatitis. Pancreatology 2002;2(6):565–573.

33. Alfandre DJ. 'I'm going home': discharges against medical advice. Mayo Clin Proc 2009;84(3):255–260.

34. Henson VL, Vickery DS. Patient self discharge from the emergency department: who is at risk? Emerg Med J 2005;22(7):499–501.

35. Wong JG, Clare IC, Gunn MJ, Holland AJ. Capacity to make health care decisions: its importance in clinical practice. Psychol Med 1999;29(2):437–446.

36. Ranjith G, Hotopf M. 'Refusing treatment – please see': an analysis of capacity assessments carried out by a liaison psychiatry service. J R Soc Med 2004;97(10):480–482.

Case perspectives: Una Lordan

THERAPEUTIC PERSPECTIVES

1 Cross-match or group and save?

- A cross-match involves matching blood from a donor to a recipient.
  It involves the physical defrosting of specific units of blood, e.g. 2 units.
  If these units are not used, they are wasted.
- A group and save establishes the patient's blood group and serum
  antibodies, but does not physically prepare units of blood for transfusion.
  If needed, units of blood can be prepared quickly, usually within
  20 minutes.
- In absolute emergencies 'unmatched blood' from a universal donor
  (O negative) can be transfused. However, stores of O negative are precious
  and should be conserved where possible.

UNA AND BLOOD

Una has had a significant bleed, vomiting half a litre, and has been passing
some melaena. While many doctors try to be conservative with the use of
blood products, in this instance Una has lost a considerable amount of blood
and is potentially continuing to bleed. For this reason cross-matching would
be prudent.

2 Do you pass a Sengstaken–Blakemore tube?

- A Sengstaken–Blakemore tube* is an oro- or nasogastric tube* with two
  balloons, one gastric and the other oesophageal, at its distal end. When
  inflated, the balloons help to tamponade bleeding. It is only a temporary
  measure as ulceration and rupture of the oesophagus are recognised
  complications.[1]
- It can be used as a temporising device to stop gastric or oesophageal
  variceal bleeding while waiting for definitive treatment.[2]
- Una does not have history of, or any risk factors for, portal hypertension.
  As Marco has told you, she usually does not drink; this has been a short
  drinking 'binge'.

*please refer to the Definitions at the end of this Case perspective.

- Particularly given the suggestion of melaena, Una's history is suggestive of peptic ulceration.

UNA AND SENGSTAKEN–BLAKEMORE TUBE

Una's history is suggestive of peptic ulcer disease and a Sengstaken–Blakemore tube is not useful in this situation but is uncomfortable and can cause complications. Your diagnosis will be confirmed by endoscopy which will also allow you to differentiate between PUD and other causes such as a Mallory–Weiss tear. If you passed a Sengstaken tube you would have been docked points and taken off the case.

3 Do you administer platelets?

- It is recommended that platelets are not allowed to drop below 50×10^9/l in the actively bleeding patient.[3]

- A higher level of 100×10^9/l has been recommended for specific cases such as multiple trauma or central nervous system injury.[3]

- In the UK a pool of platelets is prepared from approximately 4 units of blood and can be anything from 150 to 450 ml. In storage, with gentle agitation, the platelets can last approximately 5 days but following preparation for transfusion, they must be used as soon as possible, within 24 hours.[3]

UNA AND PLATELETS

Una's platelet count is 70×10^9/l. While this is lower than normal, it is above the level at which we would transfuse platelets. Una has no risk factors, such as antiplatelet drugs, to make us suspect that her platelets may not be functioning properly. If you transfused platelets you were deducted points.

4 Diastolic murmur – do you give antibiotics or not prior to scope?

- The rate of bacteraemia* as a direct result of endoscopic procedures is small (2–5%) and the organisms involved are unlikely to cause endocarditis.[4,5]

- Bacteraemia following some specific procedures such as stricture dilation can be as high as 45%.[4] Active bleeding may also slightly increase this risk.[6]

- Also important is the underlying cardiac condition.[6]

Indications for prophylaxis are shown in the following table.

High risk	Intermediate risk
Prosthetic heart valves	Most other congenital cardiac malformations
Previous bacterial endocarditis*	Acquired valvular defects (e.g. rheumatic fever)
Surgical shunts or conduits	Hypertrophic cardiomyopathy
Complex cyanotic heart disease	Mitral valve prolapse with regurgitation or thickened valves

Prophylaxis is not recommended in the following situations.

1. Isolated secundum atrial septal defect
2. Surgical repair of atrial septal defect, ventricular septal defect or patent ductus arteriosus
3. Previous cardiac bypass graft surgery
4. Mitral valve prolapse without valvular regurgitation
5. Physiological, functional or innocent cardiac murmurs
6. Previous Kawasaki's disease* without valvular dysfunction
7. Cardiac pacemakers (intravascular and epicardial) and implanted defibrillators

A single dose of oral amoxicillin is the standard prophylactic measure 1 hour before the procedure.[6]

UNA AND ENDOCARDITIS

Una has an undefined cardiac murmur. Although it may be innocent, she requires an echocardiogram to distinguish this. As a result, it would seem prudent to protect her from even a small risk associated with bacteraemia. If you did not, you lost 1 point.

5 Inject ulcer or not?

- The features of stigmata of recent haemorrhage (SRH)[7] are shown in the following table.

Endoscopic features of SRH	Rebleeding %
Pulsatile adherent bleeding	85
Adherent clot	40
Pigmented protuberance	20
Flat blood spot on ulcer base	5–10

- There are alternatives to injection, such as bipolar diathermy and laser photocoagulation.
- However, the rate of surgery for active bleeding following photocoagulation is 40% compared to just 15% with diathermy or injection.[8] Photocoagulation also requires expensive equipment while diathermy runs the risk of full-thickness burns to tissue. For this reason many units use injection therapy preferentially.

UNA AND INJECTION

While it is an ooze rather than pulsatile bleeding, there is evidence of active bleeding and a high risk of continuous or rebleeding. For this reason an endoscopic intervention is indicated. If you did not choose to do this Cahoon would have intervened and helped you. Although it was the right decision to intervene, you were not deducted points for not injecting as this could easily have been an issue of a lack of skill. Cahoon really should have been with you.

6 Inject with what? Saline or adrenaline?

- Traditionally 1:10,000 concentration of adrenaline has been used for injection of bleeding ulcers.[9]
- There has been a suggestion that injecting normal saline may give an equal result as it causes a similar tamponade* effect. However, recent evidence appears to suggest that the initial haemostatic rate is lower in the saline group.[10]

UNA AND ADRENALINE

Although studies are ongoing, it appears that adrenaline has an advantage over normal saline and so should have been chosen in Una's case.

7 Where do you inject – edge or centre?

- The needle should be advanced into the base of the bleeding point and your assistant injects 0.5 ml of the adrenaline solution.
- If resistance is not encountered, you may be in the wrong place.
- If the bleeding does not stop, a further 0.5 ml should be injected into the same site and then the needle moved to a slightly different site and the injection repeated.[11]

8 Proton pump inhibitor infusion, once daily or stop

Evidence has existed since the mid-1990s that the proton pump inhibitors given after endoscopic treatment reduce rebleeding rates, the need for surgery and hospital stay.[12,13]

Section 2

UNA AND PPI

There is strong evidence for a benefit to a PPI infusion post endoscopic intervention and so this should have been given. If you decided not to give the infusion, you were deducted points and if you stopped it altogether, Una rebled the following night.

COMMUNICATION PERSPECTIVES

Marco's perspective

• Marco is boisterous and causing a fuss in the department.
• It is difficult for staff to work with such patients.
• He displays qualities of a bully by insisting on getting things his own way, and in the way he admits to 'making' Una keep up with his alcohol excess.

SIMPSON AND MARCO

It is difficult to deal with such patients, particularly in this case where Marco is both patient and 'relative'. Una must be your priority from the moment she becomes unwell, as her condition is immediately life threatening. Marco, although not a likeable character, is a potential source of information and so communication should be maintained. As an outsider looking in, their relationship seems potentially harmful, and while the medical problems take priority right now, this is something that should be discussed or looked into further prior to discharge.

Nurse's perspective

• The nursing staff expect whoever is performing the procedure to be able to complete it.
• They begin to get nervous when it becomes clear you need Cahoon and he is not there.

SIMPSON AND THE NURSE

You are in a difficult position. You must remain calm and think clearly, but you should not undertake to perform a procedure, such as injecting, if you are not competent to do so. Cahoon should not have left you at an important point like this. Looking for Cahoon is the right thing to do and if you are unsure what to do, you have little choice but to withdraw when Una becomes uncomfortable and wait for Cahoon.

Cahoon's perspective

• Cahoon is under considerable pressure and is juggling surgery with his boss and managing patients with you.

- His boss is quite demanding and difficult. However, as you are much junior, Cahoon uses professional discretion not to discuss this with you.
- He should not have left you alone at such an important point in the procedure.
- Your inexperience is not your fault.
- Juggling different procedures is the fault of the system and is dangerous.

SIMPSON AND CAHOON

Cahoon is under considerable pressure trying to help you and keep his boss happy by assisting in theatre. While you did not know it, his boss rang him demanding his presence in theatre. Cahoon should not have left you but equally his boss should have recognised the importance of his presence at the endoscopy.

What happened to Una?

Una made a good recovery. At repeat endoscopy her ulcer had healed well and echo demonstrated that her murmur was innocent. It transpired that she was in a physically abusive relationship with Marco. After discharge they broke up, with Una leaving the region to live with her parents.

DEFINITIONS

Oro- or nasogastric tube – a tube passed through either the nose or mouth to the stomach.

Bacteraemia – the presence of bacteria in the blood.

Endocarditis – inflammation of the endocardium or heart valves.

Kawasaki's disease – a rare acute illness of children, of unknown origin that causes acute inflammation of the vessels and endocardium. It is associated with lymphadenopathy, fever and a rash.

Tamponade – compression by external pressure.

REFERENCE LIST

1. Bauer JJ, Kreel I, Kark AE. The use of the Sengstaken–Blakemore tube for immediate control of bleeding esophageal varices. Ann Surg 1974;179(3):273–277.
2. D'Amico G, Pagliaro L, Bosch J. The treatment of portal hypertension: a meta-analytic review. Hepatology 1995;22(1):332–354.
3. British Committee for Standards in Haematology, Blood Transfusion Task Force. Guidelines for the use of platelet transfusions. Br J Haematol 2003;122(1):10–23.
4. Botoman VA, Surawicz CM. Bacteremia with gastrointestinal endoscopic procedures. Gastrointest Endosc 1986;32(5):342–346.
5. Byrne WJ, Euler AR, Campbell M, Eisenach KD. Bacteremia in children following upper gastrointestinal endoscopy or colonoscopy. J Pediatr Gastroenterol Nutr 1982;1(4):551–553.

Section 2

6. Dajani AS, Taubert KA, Wilson W, et al. Prevention of bacterial endocarditis. Recommendations by the American Heart Association. Circulation 1997;96(1):358–366.

7. British Society of Gastroenterology Endoscopy Committee. Non-variceal upper gastrointestinal haemorrhage: guidelines. Gut 2002;51(Suppl 4):iv1–iv6.

8. Steele RJ. Endoscopic haemostasis for non-variceal upper gastrointestinal haemorrhage. Br J Surg 1989;76(3):219–225.

9. Liou TC, Chang WH, Wang HY, Lin SC, Shih SC. Large-volume endoscopic injection of epinephrine plus normal saline for peptic ulcer bleeding. J Gastroenterol Hepatol 2007;22(7):996–1002.

10. Lin HJ, Perng CL, Sun IC, Tseng GY. Endoscopic haemoclip versus heater probe thermocoagulation plus hypertonic saline-epinephrine injection for peptic ulcer bleeding. Dig Liver Dis 2003;35(12):898–902.

11. Paterson-Brown S. *Core Topics in General and Emergency Surgery*. Edinburgh: Elsevier Saunders, 2009.

12. Lau JY, Sung JJ, Lee KK, et al. Effect of intravenous omeprazole on recurrent bleeding after endoscopic treatment of bleeding peptic ulcers. N Engl J Med 2000;343(5):310–316.

13. Hasselgren G, Lind T, Lundell L, et al. Continuous intravenous infusion of omeprazole in elderly patients with peptic ulcer bleeding. Results of a placebo-controlled multicenter study. Scand J Gastroenterol 1997;32(4):328–333.

Case perspectives: Regina Appleton

THERAPEUTIC PERSPECTIVES

1 Myocardial infarction

- Regina has had a non-ST elevation myocardial infarction (NSTEMI).
- Acute coronary syndrome (ACS) is a spectrum of conditions which include unstable angina (UA), NSTEMI and ST elevation MI (STEMI).
- Approximately 1.5 million patients are hospitalised every year in the United States with ACS, of which 1 million represent UA or NSTEMI.[1]
- The difference between UA and NSTEMI is the presence of biochemical markers of MI and necrosis in NSTEMI. Elevated ST segments on ECG then help to distinguish STEMI from NSTEMI.[2]
- In UA and NSTEMI, there is usually an incomplete occlusion of the lumen of a coronary vessel. It is thought that in NSTEMI microemboli released from the thrombus travel downstream into the distal myocardial vascular bed, causing a microscopic focus of necrosis resulting in a rise in the markers of infarction.[3]
- In 2000 a joint consensus document by the European Society of Cardiology and the American College of Cardiology defined the diagnosis of an acute or evolving myocardial infarction as either one of the following two criteria[4]:
  1. Typical rise and gradual fall (troponin) or more rapid rise and fall (CK-MB) of biochemical markers of myocardial necrosis with at least one of the following.
     – Ischaemic symptoms
     – Development of pathological Q waves on the ECG
     – ECG changes indicative of ischaemia (ST segment elevation or depression)
     – Coronary artery intervention (e.g. coronary angioplasty)
  2. Pathological findings of an acute MI.

REGINA AND MI

Regina is a smoker with known peripheral vascular disease. She has had chest pain, has inverted T-waves on her lateral leads and a positive troponin without a rise in her ST segments. By definition, she has had a NSTEMI.

*please refer to the Definitions at the end of this Case perspective.

2 ECG

- A 12-lead ECG should be obtained within 10 minutes of presentation of patients with ongoing pain and as quickly as possible in all other patients with potential ACS.[5]
- Deep precordial T-wave inversions greater than or equal to 0.2 mV (2 mm) predict a poorer prognosis and may reflect a critical stenosis of the left anterior descending coronary artery.[6]
- It should, however, be borne in mind that a normal ECG does not exclude an infarct.[7]

REGINA AND ECG

Regina has symptoms and changes on her ECG. The tracing demonstrates inversion of the T-waves in her lateral leads, which as mentioned above may carry a poorer prognosis.

3 Cardiac enzymes

- The most widely used cardiac enzymes are creatine kinase (CK-MB) and troponins, with the troponins being the test of choice, able to detect small areas of necrosis missed by CK.[2]
- Troponins first appear 4–12 hours after the onset of symptoms.[8]
- As release may be delayed, if negative, troponins and CK should be rechecked at 8–12 hours post symptoms.[5]
- The patient's risk of death or a further MI is increased proportionally to the quantity of troponin measured.[9,10]
- Twenty-five percent of patients with elevated CK and troponin will go on to develop a STEMI.[11]

REGINA AND CARDIAC ENZYMES

Regina has a positive troponin and a raised CK. The troponin has risen earlier and suggests a significant cardiac event, distinguishing this case of NSTEMI from UA.

4 Treatment

AGENTS TO HELP LIMIT ISCHAEMIA

Oxygen

Although administered widely, oxygen has never been shown to reduce morbidity or mortality. The ACC/AHA guidelines recommend that it be administered to those patients with hypoxaemia or respiratory compromise, aiming for a saturation above 90%.

Nitrates

- Nitrates cause venodilation,* thus reducing preload. This in turn should help to reduce ventricular stress and thus oxygen demand. Nitrates also have a small effect on afterload by dilating the arterial system, including the coronary arteries, and thus improving oxygen delivery.[5]
- Despite these potential benefits, nitrates remain somewhat controversial with one review of several small studies[12] suggesting an improved survival with nitrate use, but other larger randomised controlled trials refuting this.[13,14]
- The ACC/AHA guidelines recommend that sublingual nitrates be given to the symptomatic patient. If this fails to relieve the chest pain this can be switched to intravenous nitrates.

Morphine

- Morphine can help reduce pain and anxiety, but very few studies have specifically examined its effect on patient prognosis following MI.[2]
- Currently the ACC/AHA guidelines recommend morphine for those patients with persistent pain despite nitrates or those with marked anxiety.

Beta-blockers

- By reducing heart rate and contractility, beta-blockers can decrease oxygen demands of the heart and increase diastolic time, thus increasing coronary perfusion time.[2]
- Evidence in studies looking at STEMI suggests that beta-blockers reduce mortality.[15]
- For this reason the ACC/AHA guidelines recommend early commencement of beta-blockade if there is no contraindication.

Calcium channel blockers

- These agents decrease the influx of calcium across the membranes of cardiac and smooth muscle.[2]
- While it was often thought that relaxing smooth muscle with nifedipine may help in the setting of a NSTEMI, this agent is no longer recommended (except under certain circumstances) as it causes a rapid drop in blood pressure and activation of the sympathetic system.[5]
- Conversely, the agents verapamil and diltiazem may be beneficial in patients in whom a beta-blocker is contraindicated and who do not have left ventricular dysfunction.[5]

ACE inhibitors

- Several studies have shown an improved mortality and morbidity with ACE inhibitors after MI, especially in diabetics[16] and patients with left ventricular dysfunction.[17]
- The ACC/AHA guidelines recommend that an ACE inhibitor should be used in these groups of patients.

ANTIPLATELETS

Aspirin

- In patients with NSTEMI or UA, aspirin produces a 49% risk reduction in the progression to death or MI.[5]
- The ACC/AHA guidelines recommend that patients should have non-enteric coated aspirin as soon as possible[5] if there are no contraindications such as active bleeding, severe untreated hypertension and active peptic ulcer disease.

Clopidogrel

- There is evidence that the addition of clopidogrel to aspirin in patients with NSTEMI improves patient outcomes.[18]
- However, there was also a higher rate of major bleeding, particularly in those who underwent surgery within the first 5 days of its discontinuation.[18]
- The ACC/AHA guidelines recommend that clopidogrel should be given in addition to aspirin in patients with NSTEMI if they are not at high risk of bleeding.

ANTITHROMBOTICS

Heparin

- The administration of UH reduces mortality and morbidity by approximately 50%.[5]
- Low molecular weight heparin also reduces mortality and morbidity,[19] with some evidence that LMWH is superior to UH.[20]
- The ACC/AHA guidelines recommend that either UH or LMWH should be administered to patients with NSTEMI.
- Low molecular weight heparin should not be given within 24 hours of CABG.[2]

Thrombolysis

- Thrombolysis increases the risk of death and MI when administered to patients with NSTEMI.[21,22]
- For this reason the ACC/AHA guidelines do not recommend its administration to patients unless they have indications such as:
  - Acute ST segment elevation
  - New left bundle branch block
  - A true posterior MI.

REGINA AND CARDIAC TREATMENT

Non-enteric coated aspirin will be absorbed quicker from the buccal mucosa when chewed and so should be given by this route. Regina's oxygen saturations are quite good and although often given and advised, supplemental oxygen is not essential and so you were not deducted points for not prescribing it. Regina is not in any pain and so nitrates or morphine are not indicated.

Although, as it transpired, clopidogrel may make the risk of bleeding in theatre higher, you were not to know this when you were asked to decide on administering the drug. However, it is important to make a decision regarding any potential revascularisation before administering a loading dose of clopidogrel, so in this instance it would have been important to seek the opinion of your cardiologist first. Ultimately, if a decision is taken at angiography to undertake angioplasty +/- stenting, a loading dose of clopidogrel can be given at that stage.

In addition to aspirin, a beta-blocker should also be administered. As this is not a STEMI (and Regina is 12 days post major vascular surgery), thrombolysis is potentially very dangerous and so if you tried to administer it, Ubeki rightly stepped in to suggest getting Cahoon's opinion. Ignoring her advice would have resulted in you going home early. As Regina is likely to need surgery, it may be wise to use UH which is easier to reverse in bleeding (with protamine sulphate) rather than LMWH.

Section 2

5 Contact Cahoon

- When faced with the question of whether to call for senior help, there are two values which are important to junior doctors:
  - to act responsibly when dealing with patients
  - to progress and develop towards independent practice.[23]
- Junior doctors are more likely to seek senior help if:
  - multiple events are happening simultaneously
  - the presentation or pathology could potentially cause death or irreparable harm.[23]
- One of the few studies to examine this area also identifies that junior doctors were mindful of non-patient related consequences to contacting senior colleagues.[23]
- Contacting senior colleagues too often may indicate an inability to 'progress and develop' as well as potentially 'alienating' their seniors on whom their own progression depended. Also contacting senior colleagues at night may render them tired and less effective the following day.[23]
- Stewart[23] also identifies that while textbook and personal knowledge are important, the local unwritten rules or 'cultural knowledge' are equally important. For example, 'seniors must always be kept informed', 'contact the most immediate senior first' or 'examine and assess the patient before asking for senior input'.

• The study also identifies contributory factors that might impede contacting a senior, such as a lack of confidence in the senior or a physical difficulty in locating/contacting them.

CONTACTING CAHOON

Had you decided to thrombolyse Regina, there was clearly a deficit in 'textbook' knowledge as discussed above. Furthermore, although alerted by Ubeki, if you decided to proceed regardless, you were ignoring the fact that your actions could have caused 'death or irreparable harm'. Sacrificing this to a desire to demonstrate to your senior colleagues that you can manage patients independently is completely unacceptable. Furthermore, doing so will only flag you as 'dangerous' to your colleagues, ultimately defeating your initial motivation. While all of us want to act independently and impress those senior to us, this must always take second place to the safety of our patients. When in doubt, ring your boss, and remember that these factors are what influence your juniors ringing you. Just consider, if they're out of their depth, what would you want your juniors to do?

6 Heparin

Heparin should be started as soon as possible to prevent thrombus propagation and extension of ischaemia. Unfractionated heparin* is preferred as it allows for easier reversal in potential interventions.[24]

REGINA AND HEPARIN

Regina will benefit from heparin for both her cardiac and lower limb pathology. It should have been started as soon as possible and if this was not done, you were docked points. Furthermore, as it is likely that you will need to intervene, you should have used unfractionated (intravenous) heparin as it is easier to reverse than LMWH.* If you chose LMWH you were deducted points.

7 Peripheral angiogram

• Current guidelines advocate the major value of having angiographic information prior to intervention, as this can help dictate the therapeutic approach. However, this is with the caveat that it should only be sought if the inevitable delay can be tolerated.[24]
• CT angiography is quick, convenient and allows cross-sectional imaging. However, it does not allow intervention and if a decision is made to then go ahead and perform a formal angiography therapeutically, more contrast is needed and the risk of renal impairment is increased.[24]

REGINA AND ANGIOGRAPHY

Regina is a very quick presentation and so has not been subjected to the usual delays of an outpatient coming in from home. This provides you with some time, allowing for radiological information. Doing a CT angiogram in this instance does not lend itself to intervention and so if necessary, a formal angiogram will be required, resulting in further nephrotoxic contrast. When planning your next step, you should always consider the subsequent steps.

8 Thrombolysis versus surgery

- According to current guidelines, thrombolysis* is the therapeutic option of choice when the degree of severity allows time.[24]
- Catheter-based thrombolysis has several potential advantages including:
  1. reduced risk of endothelial trauma
  2. thrombolysis of vessels too small for embolectomy catheters
  3. gradual reperfusion as opposed to the sudden high-pressure reperfusion associated with balloon embolectomy.[24]
- Surgery is immediately indicated where there are advanced signs such as some sensory loss and muscle weakness, but the limb is still salvageable.[24]

REGINA AND THROMBOLYSIS

Regina is presenting early and has no sensory loss or muscle weakness. Although she had vascular surgery only 12 days ago, she presents a real risk for anaesthetic, even local, which may ultimately result in a bypass under general anaesthetic. On the balance of risk and benefit, thrombolysis would be the option of first choice.

9 Anaesthetic

- Surgery within 4–6 weeks of a MI may increase the perioperative risk up to fivefold[25] and regional anaesthesia (e.g. epidural or spinal) may be as dangerous as GA.
- Although local anaesthesia may not have the haemodynamic effects seen with GA, inadequate analgesic control may still stimulate pain, resulting in a stress response with tachycardia and myocardial strain.
- It should also be borne in mind that a failed embolectomy may necessitate a bypass procedure, which would not be possible under just local anaesthesia.

REGINA AND ANAESTHESIA

If you followed an operative route then eventually you were faced with the decision regarding anaesthesia. Ultimately, your anaesthetist decides that initial embolectomy will be under local anaesthetic. Deciding this from the start will have earned you points.

10 Keep her anticoagulated?

- There is a high risk of recurrent limb ischaemia in the postoperative period.[26,27]
- Current guidelines recommend that all patients should be treated with heparin in the postoperative period followed by warfarin for 3–6 months or longer. The studies are weak with regard to exactly how long treatment should continue.[24]

REGINA AND ANTICOAGULATION

Regina is at high risk of recurrent ischaemia and so should be heparinised and then switched to warfarin. Failing to do this resulted in a loss of points.

COMMUNICATION PERSPECTIVES

Anaesthetist's perspective

- There is a threat to the limb.
- The patient needs an operation.
- A general anaesthetic could be potentially fatal to this patient.
- A spinal or epidural in this setting can also carry potential risks.

SIMPSON AND THE ANAESTHETIST

Your anaesthetist does not want a patient to die while she is responsible for them. Well-used local anaesthetic will allow you access without risking the patient, although you must ensure that they are comfortable and pain free, otherwise you will put their myocardium under further strain. In truth, you should really have the operating surgeon involved in making this decision and so calling Cahoon is a good idea.

What happened to Regina?

In reality, Regina did not have a good outcome. Having suffered her MI, treatment of her leg was delayed. Due to her advanced signs, a decision was taken to operate. Intraoperatively the embolus was well organised and it was not possible to retrieve by embolectomy. At this point her lower leg was viable by a very small amount of blood being delivered via collaterals, but these were not enough to guarantee prolonged viability and so an emergency bypass had to be performed. Due to the emergency nature of this, it was necessary to put Regina under GA. She survived the operation but developed heart failure in the immediate postoperative period. She was never extubated and she died 22 hours postoperatively.

DEFINITIONS

Venodilation – increases the calibre of veins.

Unfractionated heparin – an injectable anticoagulant monitored by measuring the APTT level.

Low molecular weight heparin (LMWH) – an anticoagulant derived from heparin which is administered subcutaneously and does not require monitoring with APTT.

Thrombolysis – the breakdown of blood clots by pharmaceutical means.

REFERENCE LIST

1. Thom T, Haase N, Rosamond W, et al. Heart disease and stroke statistics – 2006 update: a report from the American Heart Association Statistics Committee and Stroke Statistics Subcommittee. Circulation 2006;113(6):e85–151.

2. Kou V, Nassisi D. Unstable angina and non-ST-segment myocardial infarction: an evidence-based approach to management. Mt Sinai J Med 2006;73(1):449–468.

3. Davies MJ. The pathophysiology of acute coronary syndromes. Heart 2000;83(3):361–366.

4. Alpert JS, Thygesen K, Antman E, Bassand JP. Myocardial infarction redefined – a consensus document of The Joint European Society of Cardiology/American College of Cardiology Committee for the redefinition of myocardial infarction. J Am Coll Cardiol 2000;36(3):959–969.

5. Braunwald E, Antman EM, Beasley JW, et al. ACC/AHA 2002 guideline update for the management of patients with unstable angina and non-ST-segment elevation myocardial infarction – summary article: a report of the American College of Cardiology/American Heart Association task force on practice guidelines (Committee on the Management of Patients With Unstable Angina). J Am Coll Cardiol 2002;40(7):1366–1374.

6. de Zwaan C, Bar FW, Janssen JH, et al. Angiographic and clinical characteristics of patients with unstable angina showing an ECG pattern indicating critical narrowing of the proximal LAD coronary artery. Am Heart J 1989;117(3):657–665.

7. Rouan GW, Lee TH, Cook EF, Brand DA, Weisberg MC, Goldman L. Clinical characteristics and outcome of acute myocardial infarction in patients with initially normal or nonspecific electrocardiograms (a report from the Multicenter Chest Pain Study). Am J Cardiol 1989;64(18):1087–1092.

8. Wu AH, Apple FS, Gibler WB, Jesse RL, Warshaw MM, Valdes R Jr. National Academy of Clinical Biochemistry Standards of Laboratory Practice: recommendations for the use of cardiac markers in coronary artery diseases. Clin Chem 1999;45(7):1104–1121.

9. Antman EM, Tanasijevic MJ, Thompson B, et al. Cardiac-specific troponin I levels to predict the risk of mortality in patients with acute coronary syndromes. N Engl J Med 1996;335(18):1342–1349.

10. Lindahl B, Toss H, Siegbahn A, Venge P, Wallentin L. Markers of myocardial damage and inflammation in relation to long-term mortality in unstable coronary artery disease. FRISC Study Group. Fragmin during Instability in Coronary Artery Disease. N Engl J Med 2000;343(16):1139–1147.

11. Anderson JL, Adams CD, Antman EM, et al. ACC/AHA 2007 guidelines for the management of patients with unstable angina/non-ST-elevation myocardial infarction: a report of the American College of Cardiology/American Heart Association Task Force on Practice Guidelines (Writing Committee to Revise the 2002 Guidelines for the Management of Patients With Unstable Angina/Non-ST-Elevation Myocardial Infarction) developed in collaboration with the American College of Emergency Physicians, the Society for Cardiovascular Angiography and Interventions, and the Society of Thoracic Surgeons endorsed by the American Association of Cardiovascular and Pulmonary Rehabilitation and the Society for Academic Emergency Medicine. J Am Coll Cardiol 2007;50(7):e1–e157.

12. Yusuf S, Collins R, MacMahon S, Peto R. Effect of intravenous nitrates on mortality in acute myocardial infarction: an overview of the randomised trials. Lancet 1988;1(8594):1088–1092.

13. ISIS-4 (Fourth International Study of Infarct Survival) Collaborative Group. ISIS-4: a randomised factorial trial assessing early oral captopril, oral mononitrate, and intravenous magnesium sulphate in 58,050 patients with suspected acute myocardial infarction. Lancet 1995;345(8951):669–685.

14. Gruppo Italiano per lo Studio della Sopravvivenza nell'infarto Miocardico. GISSI-3: effects of lisinopril and transdermal glyceryl trinitrate singly and together on 6-week mortality and ventricular function after acute myocardial infarction. Lancet 1994;343(8906):1115–1122.

15. ISIS-1 (First International Study of Infarct Survival) Collaborative Group. Mechanisms for the early mortality reduction produced by beta-blockade started early in acute myocardial infarction: ISIS-1. Lancet 1988;1(8591):921–923.

16. Gustafsson I, Torp-Pedersen C, Kober L, Gustafsson F, Hildebrandt P. Effect of the angiotensin-converting enzyme inhibitor trandolapril on mortality and morbidity in diabetic patients with left ventricular dysfunction after acute myocardial infarction. Trace Study Group. J Am Coll Cardiol 1999;34(1):83–89.

17. Pfeffer MA, Braunwald E, Moye LA, et al. Effect of captopril on mortality and morbidity in patients with left ventricular dysfunction after myocardial infarction. Results of the survival and ventricular enlargement trial. The SAVE Investigators. N Engl J Med 1992;327(10):669–677.

18. Yusuf S, Zhao F, Mehta SR, Chrolavicius S, Tognoni G, Fox KK. Effects of clopidogrel in addition to aspirin in patients with acute coronary syndromes without ST-segment elevation. N Engl J Med 2001;345(7):494–502.

19. Antman EM, Cohen M, Radley D, et al. Assessment of the treatment effect of enoxaparin for unstable angina/non-Q-wave myocardial infarction. TIMI 11B-ESSENCE meta-analysis. Circulation 1999;100(15):1602–1608.

20. Antman EM, Cohen M, McCabe C, Goodman SG, Murphy SA, Braunwald E. Enoxaparin is superior to unfractionated heparin for preventing clinical events at 1-year follow-up of TIMI 11B and ESSENCE. Eur Heart J 2002;23(4):308–314.

21. No authors listed. Effects of tissue plasminogen activator and a comparison of early invasive and conservative strategies in unstable angina and non-Q-wave myocardial infarction. Results of the TIMI IIIB Trial. Thrombolysis in Myocardial Ischemia. Circulation 1994;89(4):1545–1556.

22. Schreiber TL, Rizik D, White C, et al. Randomized trial of thrombolysis versus heparin in unstable angina. Circulation 1992;86(5):1407–1414.

23. Stewart J. To call or not to call: a judgement of risk by pre-registration house officers. Med Educ 2008;42(9):938–944.

24. Norgren L, Hiatt WR, Dormandy JA, et al. Inter-Society Consensus for the Management of Peripheral Arterial Disease (TASC II). Eur J Vasc Endovasc Surg 2007;33(Suppl 1):S1–75.

25. Chassot PG, Delabays A, Spahn DR. Preoperative evaluation of patients with, or at risk of, coronary artery disease undergoing non-cardiac surgery. Br J Anaesth 2002;89(5):747–759.

26. Ouriel K, Veith FJ, Sasahara AA. A comparison of recombinant urokinase with vascular surgery as initial treatment for acute arterial occlusion of the legs. Thrombolysis or Peripheral Arterial Surgery (TOPAS) Investigators. N Engl J Med 1998;338(16):1105–1111.

27. No authors listed. Results of a prospective randomized trial evaluating surgery versus thrombolysis for ischemia of the lower extremity. The STILE trial. Ann Surg 1994;220(3):251–266.

Section 2

Case perspectives: Susie Redback

THERAPEUTIC PERSPECTIVES

1 Radiology

• Your number one differential should be gallstones.

• Standard ultrasound has a sensitivity in excess of 95% for gallstones.[1]

• As Susie's symptoms and signs have completely resolved, it is possible to distinguish between cholelithiasis* and cholecystitis.* Ultrasonography also has the ability to radiologically distinguish between these two conditions.[2]

• It is estimated that only about 15% of gallstones are calcified enough to be seen on plain films.[3]

• Computed tomography has been shown to have a limited sensitivity of 79% for the detection of uncomplicated gallstones.[4] However, this is still an evolving technique, with some researchers estimating the sensitivity to be higher than this.

SUSIE AND RADIOLOGY

Examination allows for a focused, cost-effective use of radiology. You were docked marks because of this, if you ordered radiology before examining Susie. Furthermore, the optimum manner in which to visualise gallstones is with ultrasound. If you chose a plain film you would have failed to see the gallstone and were deducted points. If you tried to book a CT for this reason, the radiologist would have changed your request to the radiation-free ultrasound, and you were deducted points.

2 Weight and surgery

• The World Health Organization (WHO) classifies those with a BMI* of over 30 to be obese.

• Complications and concurrent medical problems are more common in the obese patient.

• The risk of atrial fibrillation increases 50% in the obese population.[5]

• Obesity is a risk factor for surgical site wound infection, possibly because of decreased oxygen tension in avascular adipose tissue[6] or immune impairment.[7] A laparoscopic approach can reduce this risk.[8]

• Obesity increases postoperative complications including pneumonia,[9] atelectasis[10] and hypoxaemia.[11]

*please refer to the Definitions at the end of this Case perspective.

- Some studies have claimed that obesity as a major risk factor for surgery may be an exaggeration.[12]
- There has been some criticism of studies looking at obesity, particularly with regard to the many ways in which obesity can be defined.[13]

SUSIE AND OBESITY

While there is some controversy over the exact impact of obesity on surgical outcomes, there is enough evidence to show that obese patients are more likely to suffer complications. Susie is facing an elective procedure and has the opportunity to reduce her weight, potentially helping her surgery and improving her overall health. Although your position in the emergency department is to treat specific illness, you have a responsibility to improve the overall health of your patient and in this case help her safely through the surgery you have planned. You were deducted marks if you did not take this opportunity.

3 Smoking and surgery

- Smoking increases postoperative complications.[14–17]
- Smoking cessation up to 4 weeks before elective surgery has been shown to reduce postoperative complications from 41% to 21%.[18–20]
- This benefit is most likely a combination of improved oxygen delivery and a reduction in the immune-modulating* effects of smoking.[18, 19]

SUSIE AND SMOKING CESSATION

Certainly, you are given the opportunity to encourage Susie to stop smoking, even for 4 weeks prior to surgery. The study quoted above by Lindstrom et al.[20] certainly demonstrated that this reduced postoperative complications. However, this group did use a smoking cessation officer and intensive programme to achieve their objectives. This type of adjunct is almost definitely necessary to reproduce their results. Apart from the short-term gain of reducing postoperative complications, this strategy has far-reaching public health implications as it appears that those who stop smoking in the preoperative period are more likely than others to stay off cigarettes.[20,21] You should have used this opportunity with Susie to encourage her to stop smoking and provided her with the necessary supports.

4 OCP and surgery

- Difficult issue with poor evidence.
- Even the low-dose OCP results in a three- to sixfold increased risk of venous thromboembolism (VTE).[22]* This risk is highest in the first year of use, but there is a persistent risk with long-term use.[23]

- Abdominal surgery increases the risk of thromboembolism by creating a hypercoagulable state.[24]
- The use of LMWH reduces the risk of thromboembolism.[25] However, the optimal duration of therapy remains controversial.
- Oral contraceptive pill use results in an increase in the coagulation factors fibrinogen and factor X and a reduction in antithrombin III, which is not balanced by an increase in protein C or plasminogen levels. This combination is potentially prothrombotic.[26]
- The result of the risks mentioned above has been a recommendation by some authors that the OCP should be stopped 4 weeks before surgery.[26] However, this is an area which requires more randomised data, including the use of LMWH to offset OCP risk.

SUSIE AND STOPPING THE OCP

While stopping the OCP preoperatively is the choice of many surgeons, the data in this area are poor. Certainly, there exists evidence that both abdominal surgery and the OCP increase the risk of VTE, and intuitively, stopping the OCP should reduce this risk. For this reason, if you did not advise Susie to stop the OCP you were not deducted points. However, Cahoon would have become upset as it was his personal practice as the operating surgeon to stop it.

COMMUNICATION PERSPECTIVES

Cahoon's perspective

- Cahoon is answerable to his own senior colleague.
- Delays in theatre are disruptions to the service.
- He is anxious to minimise any possible complications in those patients on whom he is operating.

SIMPSON AND CAHOON

If you failed to take advantage of the opportunity to reduce Susie's risk profile, Cahoon became upset and angry. This resulted in you being deducted marks. You should take every opportunity to reduce the morbidity and mortality of your patients.

Susie's perspective

- Susie is pain free.
- Susie is asymptomatic but stuck in an emergency department alone.

• She is anxious to attend a reception and her presence in the emergency department is delaying her.

SIMPSON AND SUSIE

You must focus on what needs to be done. In this scenario it is difficult as the patient does not know what is wrong but is happy that her symptoms have gone. She is angry that it is detracting from her social commitments. If you failed to follow up Susie in the community, she would have re-presented with a life-threatening pancreatitis, and while this may be rare, it emphasises the importance of appropriate follow-up where it is needed.

What happened to Susie?

Susie returned 6 weeks later for an elective cholecystectomy. Her gallbladder was quite stuck and the procedure difficult. Susie was kept overnight and made a good recovery. She complained of mild pain in her right shoulder for about 48 hours after surgery. This was a result of gas from the pneumoperitoneum irritating her diaphragm. This resolved spontaneously and Susie made a full recovery.

DEFINITIONS

Cholelithiasis – gallstones.

Cholecystitis – inflammation of the gallbladder.

BMI (BMI) – body weight (kg)/height^2 (metres).

Immune modulating – altering the normal functioning of the immune system with a view to improving its performance.

Venous thromboembolism – the formation of a blood clot within the lumen of a vein.

REFERENCE LIST

1. Cooperberg PL, Gibney RG. Imaging of the gallbladder, 1987. Radiology 1987;163(3):605–613.

2. Soyer P, Brouland JP, Boudiaf M, et al. Color velocity imaging and power Doppler sonography of the gallbladder wall: a new look at sonographic diagnosis of acute cholecystitis. AJR 1998;171(1):183–188.

3. Stein JH. *Internal Medicine*. Philadelphia: Elsevier Health Sciences, 1998.

4. Barakos JA, Ralls PW, Lapin SA, et al. Cholelithiasis: evaluation with CT. Radiology 1987;162(2):415–418.

5. Wang TJ, Parise H, Levy D, et al. Obesity and the risk of new-onset atrial fibrillation. JAMA 2004;292(20):2471–2477.

6. Dindo D, Muller MK, Weber M, Clavien PA. Obesity in general elective surgery. Lancet 2003;361(9374):2032–2035.

7. Tanaka S, Inoue S, Isoda F, et al. Impaired immunity in obesity: suppressed but reversible lymphocyte responsiveness. Int J Obes Relat Metab Disord 1993;17(11):631–636.

8. Nguyen NT, Goldman C, Rosenquist CJ, et al. Laparoscopic versus open gastric bypass: a randomized study of outcomes, quality of life, and costs. Ann Surg 2001;234(3):279–289.

9. Brooks-Brunn JA. Predictors of postoperative pulmonary complications following abdominal surgery. Chest 1997;111(3):564–571.

10. Eichenberger A, Proietti S, Wicky S, et al. Morbid obesity and postoperative pulmonary atelectasis: an underestimated problem. Anesth Analg 2002;95(6):1788–1792.

11. Jackson CV. Preoperative pulmonary evaluation. Arch Intern Med 1988;148(10):2120–2127.

12. Dindo D, Muller MK, Weber M, Clavien PA. Obesity in general elective surgery. Lancet 2003;361(9374):2032–2035.

13. Gendall KA, Raniga S, Kennedy R, Frizelle FA. The impact of obesity on outcome after major colorectal surgery. Dis Colon Rectum 2007;50(12):2223–2237.

14. Myles PS, Iacono GA, Hunt JO, et al. Risk of respiratory complications and wound infection in patients undergoing ambulatory surgery: smokers versus nonsmokers. Anesthesiology 2002;97(4):842–847.

15. Finan KR, Vick CC, Kiefe CI, Neumayer L, Hawn MT. Predictors of wound infection in ventral hernia repair. Am J Surg 2005;190(5):676–681.

16. Selber JC, Kurichi JE, Vega SJ, Sonnad SS, Serletti JM. Risk factors and complications in free TRAM flap breast reconstruction. Ann Plast Surg 2006;56(5):492–497.

17. Sorensen LT, Hemmingsen U, Kallehave F, et al. Risk factors for tissue and wound complications in gastrointestinal surgery. Ann Surg 2005;241(4):654–658.

18. Panagiotakos DB, Pitsavos C, Chrysohoou C, et al. Effect of exposure to secondhand smoke on markers of inflammation: the ATTICA study. Am J Med 2004;116(3):145–150.

19. Greif R, Akca O, Horn EP, Kurz A, Sessler DI. Supplemental perioperative oxygen to reduce the incidence of surgical-wound infection. Outcomes Research Group. N Engl J Med 2000;342(3):161–167.

20. Lindstrom D, Sadr AO, Wladis A, et al. Effects of a perioperative smoking cessation intervention on postoperative complications: a randomized trial. Ann Surg 2008;248(5):739–745.

21. Moller A, Villebro N. Interventions for preoperative smoking cessation. Cochrane Database Syst Rev 2005;3:CD002294.

22. Venous thromboembolic disease and combined oral contraceptives: results of international multicentre case-control study. World Health Organization Collaborative Study of Cardiovascular Disease and Steroid Hormone Contraception. Lancet 1995;346(8990):1575–1582.

23. Herings RM, Urquhart J, Leufkens HG. Venous thromboembolism among new users of different oral contraceptives. Lancet 1999;354(9173):127–128.

24. Iversen LH, Thorlacius-Ussing O. Relationship of coagulation test abnormalities to tumour burden and postoperative DVT in resected colorectal cancer. Thromb Haemost 2002;87(3):402–408.

25. Geerts WH, Heit JA, Clagett GP, et al. Prevention of venous thromboembolism. Chest 2001;119(1 Suppl):132S–175S.

26. Robinson GE, Burren T, Mackie IJ, et al. Changes in haemostasis after stopping the combined contraceptive pill: implications for major surgery. BMJ 1991;302(6771):269–271.

INVESTIGATIONS

Name: Marco Baldinelli   MRN: 109684 DOB: 18/05/1991
Adress: Apt 354 Wilcox Estate Loc: Emergency Dept.
            Sex: M Phone: Req by: Simpson
Specimen No: PH763568 (Haematology)   <PgDn> for later samples

PH763568	12/03/2011	21:50	Whole Blood			
WBC	18.3	$\times10^9$/L	(	4 to 11	)	Auth
RBC	5.2	$\times10^{12}$/l	(	4.5 to 5.3	)	Auth
HB	14.2	g/dl	(	12 to 16	)	Auth
HCT	0.52	l/l	(	0.36 to 0.5	)	Auth
MCV	95.5	fl	(	76 to 96	)	Auth
MCH	28.0	pg	(	27 to 32	)	Auth
MCHC	35.5	g/dl	(	32 to 36	)	Auth
PLT	450	$\times10^9$/1	(	140 to 440	)	Auth
Neutrophils	12.60	$\times10^9$/l	(	1.8 to 8	)	Auth
Lymphocytes	3.90	$\times10^9$/l	(	1.5 to 3.5	)	Auth
Monocytes	0.94	$\times10^9$/l	(	0.16 to 1	)	Auth
Eosinophils	0.43	$\times10^9$/l	(	0 to 0.5	)	Auth
Basophils	0.13	$\times10^9$/l	(	0 to 0.2	)	Auth
INR	1.0		(	1 to 1.2	)	Auth
APTT	30	SEC	(	22 to 30	)	Auth

1 Date 2 Earlst 3 Latst 4 rep seQ 5 Spec 6 DFT 7 Matches 8 Options 9 Exit X
        No more samples
Disc: HAEM Sect: Haem Pilgrims Emergency department WRNQ/APEX
Overtype

Name: Marco Baldinelli   MRN: 109684 DOB: 18/05/1991
Adress: Apt 354 Wilcox Estate Loc: Emergency Dept. Pilgrims
            Sex: M Phone: Req by: Simpson
Specimen No: PH763522 (Biochemistry)   <PgDn> for later samples

PH763522	12/03/2011	21:50	Whole Blood		
Sodium	148	mmol/L	(132 to 144	)	Auth
Potassium	4.8	mmol/L	(3.5 to 5.0	)	Auth
Chloride	100	mmol/L	(95 to 107	)	Auth
Urea	11.0	mmol/L	(2.5 to 7.0	)	Auth
Creatinine	120	umol/L	(50 to 130	)	Auth
Total Protein	80	g/L	(62 to 82	)	Auth
Albumin	42	g/L	(36 to 44	)	Auth
AST	150	U/L	(6 to 42	)	Auth
ALT	90	U/L	(4 to 45	)	Auth
Total Bilirubin	28	umol/L	(2 to 20	)	Auth
GGT	450	U/L	(6 to 48	)	Auth
Alkaline Phosphatase	180	U/L	(40 to 130	)	Auth
Amylase	1203	U/L	(28 to 150	)	Auth
C-Reactive Protein	134	mg/l	(0 to 10	)	Auth
Calcium	2.5	mmol/L	(2.1 to 2.62	)	Auth
Haemolysis index	0				

1 Date 2 Earlst 3 Latst 4 rep seQ 5 Spec 6 DFT 7 Matches 8 Options 9 Exit X
Disc: Biochem Sect: Biochem Pilgrims Emergency department WRNQ/APEX
Overtype

Name: Marco Baldinelli   MRN: 109684   DOB: 18/05/1991
Adress: Apt 354 Wilcox Estate   Loc: Emergency Dept. Pilgrims
                                        Sex: M   Phone: Req by: Simpson
Specimen No: PH763523   (Biochemistry)   <PgDn> for later samples

PH763522	12/03/2011	21:54	Whole Blood		
pH	7.42			(7.36 to 7.44)	Auth
pCo2	4.8	kPa		(4.5 to 6.1)	Auth
po2	10.2	kPa		(11.3 to 14)	Auth
Actual bicarbonate	24	mmol/L		(22 to 26)	Auth
Base excess	1.2	mmol/L		(−2.5 to 2.5)	Auth
Oxygen saturation	92	%		( )	Auth
Lactate	2.8	mmol/L		(0 to 2)	Auth

1 Date 2 Earlst 3 Latst 4 rep seQ 5 Spec 6 DFT 7 Matches 8 Options 9 Exit X
Disc: Biochem Sect: Biochem Pilgrims Emergency department WRNQ/APEX
Overtype

Name: Una Lordan   MRN: 109681   DOB: 01/02/1992
Adress: Apt 354 Wilcox Estate   Loc: Emergency Dept. Pilgrims
                                        Sex: F   Phone: Req by: Simpson
Specimen No: PH763589   (Haematology)   <PgDn> for later samples

PH763578	12/03/2011	22:55	Whole Blood		
WBC	9.5	×10^9/L		(4 to 11)	Auth
RBC	4.5	×10^12/l		(4.5 to 5.3)	Auth
HB	13.6	g/dl		(12 to 16)	Auth
HCT	0.39	l/l		(0.36 to 0.5)	Auth
MCV	90.5	fl		(76 to 96)	Auth
MCH	30.1	pg		(27 to 32)	Auth
MCHC	34.3	g/dl		(32 to 36)	Auth
PLT	70	×10^9/l		(140 to 440)	Auth
Neutrophils	9.64	×10^9/l		(1.8 to 8)	Auth
Lymphocytes	2.30	×10^9/l		(1.5 to 3.5)	Auth
Monocytes	0.23	×10^9/l		(0.16 to 1)	Auth
Eosinophils	0.23	×10^9/l		(0 to 0.5)	Auth
Basophils	0.16	×10^9/l		(0 to 0.2)	Auth
INR	1.0			(1 to 1.2)	Auth
APTT	24	SEC		(22 to 30)	Auth

1 Date 2 Earlst 3 Latst 4 rep seQ 5 Spec 6 DFT 7 Matches 8 Options 9 Exit X
No more samples
Disc: HAEM Sect: Haem Pilgrims Emergency department WRNQ/APEX Overtype

Name: Una Lordan   MRN: 109681   DOB: 01/02/1992
Adress: Apt. 354 Wilcox estate   Loc: Emergency Dept. Pilgrims
                                    Sex: M   Phone: Req by: Simpson
Specimen No: PH763589   (Biochemistry)   <PgDn> for later samples

PH763517	12/03/2011	22:55	Whole Blood		
Sodium	139		mmol/L	(132 to 144)	Auth
Potassium	4.3		mmol/L	(3.5 to 5.0)	Auth
Chloride	93		mmol/L	(95 to 107)	Auth
Urea	9.0		mmol/L	(2.5 to 7.0)	Auth
Creatinine	86		umol/L	(50 to 130)	Auth
Total Protein	68		g/L	(62 to 82)	Auth
Amylase	90		U/L	(28 to 150)	Auth
Haemolysis index	0				

1 Date 2 Earlst 3 Latst 4 rep seQ 5 Spec 6 DFT 7 Matches 8 Options 9 Exit X
Disc: Biochem Sect: Biochem Pilgrims Emergency department WRNQ/APEX
Overtype

Name: Norma Nowak   MRN: 117844   DOB: 09/03/1939
Adress: 287 Sunny Vale   Loc: Emergency Dept. Pilgrims
        MacAuliffe Meadows   Sex: F   Phone: Req by: Simpson
Specimen No: PH763598   (Haematology)   <PgDn> for later samples

PH763517	12/03/2011	23:10	Whole Blood		
WBC	7.2		×10^9/L	(4 to 11)	Auth
RBC	4.28		×10^12/l	(4.5 to 5.3)	Auth
HB	12.9		g/dl	(12 to 16)	Auth
HCT	0.42		l/l	(0.36 to 0.5)	Auth
MCV	90.5		fl	(76 to 96)	Auth
MCH	30.0		pg	(27 to 32)	Auth
MCHC	35.7		g/dl	(32 to 36)	Auth
PLT	180		×10^9/l	(140 to 440)	Auth
Neutrophils	3.80		×10^9/l	(1.8 to 8)	Auth
Lymphocytes	1.40		×10^9/l	(1.5 to 3.5)	Auth
Monocytes	0.84		×10^9/l	(0.16 to 1)	Auth
Eosinophils	0.36		×10^9/l	(0 to 0.5)	Auth
Basophils	0.11		×10^9/l	(0 to 0.2)	Auth

1 Date 2 Earlst 3 Latst 4 rep seQ 5 Spec 6 DFT 7 Matches 8 Options 9 Exit X
No more samples
Disc: HAEM Sect: Haem Pilgrims Emergency department WRNQ/APEX Overtype

Section 2

Name: Norma Nowak   MRN: 117844   DOB: 09/03/1939
Adress: 287 Sunny Vale   Loc: Emergency Dept. Pilgrims
       MacAuliffe Meadows   Sex: F   Phone: Req by: Simpson
Specimen No: PH763623   (Biochemistry)   <PgDn> for later samples

PH763534	12/03/2011	01:10	Whole Blood		
Sodium	136	mmol/L	(132 to 144)	Auth
Potassium	3.9	mmol/L	(3.5 to 5.0)	Auth
Chloride	100	mmol/L	(95 to 107)	Auth
Urea	4.0	mmol/L	(2.5 to 7.0)	Auth
Creatinine	59	umol/L	(50 to 130)	Auth
C-Reactive Protein	1	mg/L	(0 to 10)	Auth
Haemolysis index	0			

1 Date 2 Earlst 3 Latst 4 rep seQ 5 Spec 6 DFT 7 Matches 8 Options 9 Exit X
Disc: Biochem Sect: Biochem Pilgrims Emergency department WRNQ/APEX
Overtype

Name: Susie Redback   MRN: 109682   DOB: 22/07/1977
Adress: 1 Dooleys Wood   Loc: Emergency Dept. Pilgrims
     Sex: F   Phone: Req by: Simpson
Specimen No: PH763590   (Haematology)   <PgDn> for later samples

PH763517	13/03/2011	01:10	Whole Blood		
WBC	8.2	x10^9/L	(4 to 11)	Auth
RBC	4.88	x10^12/l	(4.5 to 5.3)	Auth
HB	12.2	g/dl	(12 to 16)	Auth
HCT	0.41	l/l	(0.36 to 0.5)	Auth
MCV	91.5	fl	(76 to 96)	Auth
MCH	30.0	pg	(27 to 32)	Auth
MCHC	35.3	g/dl	(32 to 36)	Auth
PLT	78	x10^9/l	(140 to 440)	Auth
Neutrophils	4.80	x10^9/l	(1.8 to 8)	Auth
Lymphocytes	1.30	x10^9/l	(1.5 to 3.5)	Auth
Monocytes	0.64	x10^9/l	(0.16 to 1)	Auth
Eosinophils	0.26	x10^9/l	(0 to 0.5)	Auth
Basophils	0.01	x10^9/l	(0 to 0.2)	Auth
INR	1.0		(1 to 1.2)	Auth
APTT	26	SEC	(22 to 30)	Auth

1 Date 2 Earlst 3 Latst 4 rep seQ 5 Spec 6 DFT 7 Matches 8 Options 9 Exit X
No more samples
Disc: HAEM Sect: Haem Pilgrims Emergency department WRNQ/APEX Overtype

Name: Susie Redback　　　　　MRN: 109682　　　DOB: 22/07/1977
Adress: 1 Dooleys wood　　　　Loc: Emergency Dept. Pilgrims
　　　　　　　　　　　　　　Sex: F　Phone:　　　Req by: Simpson
Specimen No: PH763534　(Biochemistry)　　　<PgDn> for later samples

PH763534	12/03/2011	01:10	Whole Blood		
Sodium	133	mmol/L	(132 to 144)	Auth
Potassium	3.6	mmol/L	(3.5 to 5.0)	Auth
Chloride	98	mmol/L	(95 to 107)	Auth
Urea	3.0	mmol/L	(2.5 to 7.0)	Auth
Creatinine	54	umol/L	(50 to 130)	Auth
Total Protein	70	g/L	(62 to 82)	Auth
Albumin	43	g/L	(36 to 44)	Auth
AST	40	U/L	(6 to 42)	Auth
ALT	32	U/L	(4 to 45)	Auth
Total Bilirubin	15	umol/L	(2 to 20)	Auth
GGT	42	U/L	(6 to 48)	Auth
Alkaline Phosphatase	102	U/L	(40 to 130)	Auth
Amylase	34	U/L	(28 to 150)	Auth
C-Reactive Protein	5	mg/L	(0 to 10)	Auth
Calcium	2.5	mmol/L	(2.1 to 2.62)	Auth
Haemolysis index	0			

1 Date　2 Earlst　3 Latst　4 rep seQ　5 Spec　6 DFT　7 Matches　8 Options　9 Exit X
Disc: Biochem　Sect: Biochem　Pilgrims Emergency department　WRNQ/APEX
Overtype

Name: Regina Appleton　　　　　　MRN: 109683　　　DOB: 04/06/1958
Adress: The Hilltop, McCarthy's gardens Loc: Surgical Ward Pilgrims
　　　　　　　　　　　　　　　Sex: F　Phone:　　　Req by: Simpson
Specimen No: PH763578　(Haematology)　　　<PgDn> for later samples

PH763578	13/03/2011	00:17	Whole Blood		
WBC	8.9	×10^9/L	(4 to 11)	Auth
RBC	4.55	×10^12/l	(4.5 to 5.3)	Auth
HB	10.2	g/dl	(12 to 16)	Auth
HCT	0.38	l/l	(0.36 to 0.5)	Auth
MCV	92.5	fl	(76 to 96)	Auth
MCH	30.0	pg	(27 to 32)	Auth
MCHC	33.3	g/dl	(32 to 36)	Auth
PLT	189	×10^9/l	(140 to 440)	Auth
Neutrophils	4.80	×10^9/l	(1.8 to 8)	Auth
Lymphocytes	2.90	×10^9/l	(1.5 to 3.5)	Auth
Monocytes	0.84	×10^9/l	(0.16 to 1)	Auth
Eosinophils	0.23	×10^9/l	(0 to 0.5)	Auth
Basophils	0.11	×10^9/l	(0 to 0.2)	Auth
INR	1.1		(1 to 1.2)	Auth
APTT	29	SEC	(22 to 30)	Auth

1 Date　2 Earlst　3 Latst　4 rep seQ　5 Spec　6 DFT　7 Matches　8 Options　9 Exit X
　　　　　　　　　　　No more samples
Disc: HAEM　Sect: Haem　Pilgrims Emergency department　WRNQ/APEX
Overtype

Name: Regina Appleton   MRN: 109683   DOB: 04/06/1958
Adress: The Hilltop, McCarthys gardens Loc: Surgical Ward. Pilgrims
                                Sex: F   Phone: Req by: Simpson
Specimen No: PH763510   (Biochemistry)   <PgDn> for later samples

PH763510	13/03/2011	00:17	Whole Blood		
Sodium		134	mmol/L	(132 to 144)	Auth
Potassium		3.6	mmol/L	(3.5 to 5.0)	Auth
Chloride		99	mmol/L	(95 to 107)	Auth
Urea		3.0	mmol/L	(2.5 to 7.0)	Auth
Creatinine		90	umol/L	(50 to 130)	Auth
Total Protein		69	g/L	(62 to 82)	Auth
Albumin		40	g/L	(36 to 44)	Auth
AST		44	U/L	(6 to 42)	Auth
ALT		40	U/L	(4 to 45)	Auth
Total Bilirubin		16	umol/L	(2 to 20)	Auth
CK		167	U/L	(20 to 140)	Auth
Alkaline Phosphatase		104	U/L	(40 to 130)	Auth
Amylase		32	U/L	(28 to 150)	Auth
C-Reactive Protein		9	mg/L	(0 to 10)	Auth
Troponin I		3.1	ng/mL	(0 to 2.5)	Auth
Haemolysis index		0			

1 Date 2 Earlst 3 Latst 4 rep seQ 5 Spec 6 DFT 7 Matches 8 Options 9 Exit X
Disc: Biochem Sect: Biochem Pilgrims Emergency department WRNQ/APEX
Overtype

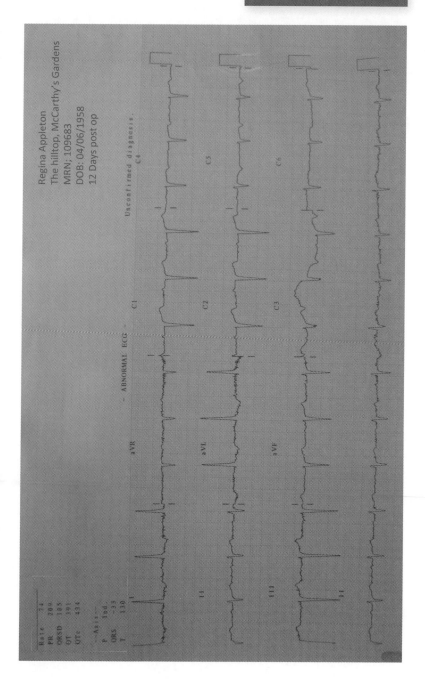

Regina Appleton
The hilltop, McCarthy's Gardens
MRN; 109683
DOB: 04/06/1958
12 Days post op

SECTION 3

What you're going to learn

After this section you will be able to manage late postoperative complications.

What you might also learn

Following completion of this section you will be capable of exhibit the following.
- A good understanding of the social implications of a patient being unwell.
- Handling difficult situations with patients and their relatives.
- The management of simple chest trauma.
- An understanding of the social and epidemiological implications of your daily decisions.

03.02 IT'S NEARLY OVER

The doctor's room is a mess, with newspapers strewn over the old tattered armchairs. The 24-hour news channel features a piece on a tiger that has escaped from his zoo enclosure and savaged three llamas. *'I know how he feels,'* grunts Cahoon from the corner of the room, sitting with his arms folded and legs outstretched. Not sure if he's joking, you laugh nervously, desperately wishing there was somebody else in the room. Cahoon looks up at you: *'How you doing, Simpson?'.* Quickly, you tell him that you're doing just fine and it's great to be here, realising how stupid that sounds at three in the morning. Cahoon smiles. *'Nobody wants to be here at three in the morning Simpson, but you're doing all right. Your first night on call isn't easy. I remember mine. I thought my boss was going to either sack me or retire. You'll be fine. There is an old patient of mine in the emergency department that I know well, so I'll drop down and see her now, and then I'm going to make sure our preops are ready for the morning. I'll talk to you later.'* For the first time, you realise that Cahoon isn't much different from you, he's just seen more years than you have. Encouraged, you look at the clock, knowing that you've nearly made it, and head back down to the department.

Downstairs, there is still no sign of the man with cellulitis and as you're calling his name the receptionist gently takes his chart from your hand. *'I don't think he's coming back, I'll file this away,'* she says softly. As you walk back to the slot, Margaret hands you a chart. *'This guy is in cubicle 3 and is refusing to see any of our emergency doctors and is insisting on seeing the surgical doctor on call.'* Knowing that by the sound of it, you're going to have to see this man sooner or later, you walk over to cubicle 3 and introduce yourself to Johnny Wassan, who is a 37-year-old father of two currently in town on business. His affect is somewhat blunted and his conversation stilted. Asking him what is wrong, he points to his lower abdomen and tells you he has some pain. Do you:

> I. *Try to take a further history* ···⟩ **409**

> II. *Examine him* ···⟩ **344**

> III. *Tell him that you're really busy and that unless he tells you what's wrong you'll go and see somebody else* ···⟩ **357**

328 Yes, you want a wide-bore tube for drainage; **add 1 point**. You carefully pass the tube and immediately aspirate 2300 ml from her stomach and instantly she feels more comfortable. What will you do next?

> I. *Give IV fluids* ···⟩ **354**

> II. *Order radiology* ···⟩ **376**

> III. *Schedule theatre* ···⟩ **403**

329 Much to Al's relief, as well as his wife's, you tell him that it should be OK to travel as long as it's more than 14 days after resolution of his pneumothorax. **Add 1 point**, and check the slot one more time.

> ···⟩ **395**

330 Yes, you want a wide-bore tube for drainage; **add 1 point**. You carefully pass the tube and immediately aspirate 2300 ml; from her stomach and instantly she feels more comfortable. What will you do next?

> I. *Nothing, observe for the moment* ···⟩ **365**

> II. *Order radiology* ···⟩ **376**

> III. *Schedule theatre* ···⟩ **403**

331 PFA of Johnny Wassan

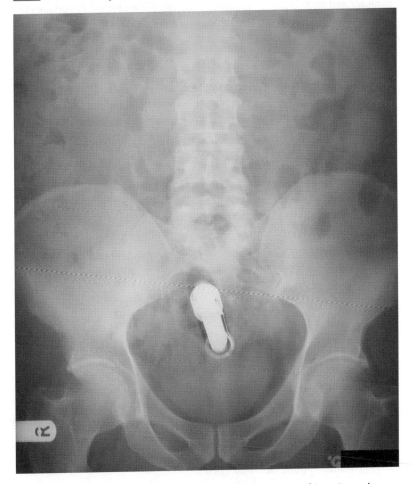

The device can be seen at the upper part of the rectum and is not causing any obvious obstruction. What would you like to do next?

I. Arrange an examination under anaesthesia ⋯⟩ **415**

II. Arrange a laparotomy and resection ⋯⟩ **383**

III. Admit and wait for it to pass ⋯⟩ **341**

IV. Discharge with instructions that it is likely to pass by itself ⋯⟩ **422**

332 You are just filling out a request when Joy observes that Lizzie is still vomiting and quite distended, asking if you think it might be a good idea to pass an NG tube before sending her down to the x-ray department? A little embarrassed, you agree. **Deduct 1 point.**

⸱⸱⸱⸱⸳ 418

333 You decide to treat the obstruction conservatively and Cahoon agrees. However, he tells you to decompress her with an NG tube, **deduct 1 point**, and asks you to get a PFA as he would like to have an idea of the level of obstruction. You do this and it shows a mid-ileal obstruction.

⸱⸱⸱⸱⸳ 337

334 Looking at the clock, it's 7.45 and your on call finishes at 8.00. You check the slot once more and it's empty. Just when you thought you had made it, Eileen calls you over to see a man with chest pain that she's worried about. Do you:

> *I. Tell Eileen that you're the surgical doctor on call, try the physician* ⸱⸱⸱⸳ **348**

> *II. Go and see the patient* ⸱⸱⸱⸳ **368**

> *III. Ask her why she thinks it's a surgical problem* ⸱⸱⸱⸳ **362**

335 You insert the nasal prongs and slowly his O_2 sats rise, which allows Al to give you a history more easily. He tells you that yesterday morning he was standing on the third step of a small ladder when he fell back and banged his chest on the rail of the stairs. He has had chest pain since but he couldn't sleep last night because he has become more breathless. Isabella grunts and turns away, muttering *'He just wants to get out of having my sister over this weekend'*. Al goes on to tell you that he does not have any real medical problems. Having taken the history, you switch him to oxygen through a face mask and examine him. **Add 1 point**.

⸱⸱⸱⸱⸳ 390

336 What will you put on the radiology form for clinical examination findings?

> *I. Make it up* ⸱⸱⸱⸳ **420**

> *II. Leave it blank* ⸱⸱⸱⸳ **346**

> *III. Reconsider and examine first* ⸱⸱⸱⸳ **361**

337 You tell Lizzie that adhesions are the most likely explanation for her bowel obstruction. She is very upset and wants to know if she should cancel her wedding in 6 days time. What will you tell her?

I. Yes ⋯⟫ **416**

II. No ⋯⟫ **421**

338 You perform a postprocedure sigmoidoscopy to ensure there is no damage and everything looks fine; **add 1 point**.

⋯⟫ **425**

339 You ring Ruth and discuss the case with her. She cannot understand how a CT will change your management tonight, and feels that if you wanted to know the level of obstruction then you should have first got a plain film. You try to make your point but there's no arguing with her. You order your plain film.

⋯⟫ **406**

340 You add potassium to her fluids. **Add 1 point**. Her abdomen is distended and tympanic but is not tender. You can feel the staple line on rectal examination and it admits your digit with ease and no obvious stricture. She has no hernia. What will you do next?

I. Order radiology ⋯⟫ **332**

II. Pass an NG tube ⋯⟫ **418**

III. Organise theatre ⋯⟫ **403**

IV. Nothing, observe for the moment ⋯⟫ **333**

341 The next morning, Cahoon is rounding and wants to know how you expected this thing to pass. *'It's certainly not obstructing, Simpson, but hey, that ain't going to come down on its own. We'll schedule an examination under anaesthesia and see if we can get it out.'*

⋯⟫ **401**

342 Much to their disappointment, you tell him that there's no way they'll be able to travel. *'Typical,'* Isabella mutters. They cancel their holiday the following day but when they try to claim the insurance, the company tells them that there is no medical reason why they couldn't have travelled. The whole thing turns into an awful mess and Halsted ends up in the middle of it. **Deduct 1 point**, and check the slot one more time.

⋯⟫ **395**

343 Good idea; **add 1 point**.

⋯⟩ **331**

344 You should always focus your examination with a history first; **deduct 1 point**. You gently begin to palpate his abdomen. Placing your hand over his umbilicus, you feel a slow gentle buzzing. Baffled, it takes you a few seconds to realise what has happened.

⋯⟩ **424**

345 You give Al oxygen by face mask and it slowly brings up his saturations. Turning to his wife Isabella, you ask her what happened. She continues to look away and tells you, *'He was supposed to put up the wallpaper yesterday because my sister, who I haven't seen in a year, is staying with us for a week from tomorrow. I asked him to do one thing and he makes a mess of it'*. You try to get her back on track by asking exactly what happened but she is dismissive. *'He says he fell and hit his chest, but he hates her, you know, hates her, I remember our wedding day, it was pouring rain and the car…'* Knowing you're not getting anywhere, you politely cut her off and try take a history from Al. It is difficult with the mask on but he manages to tell you that he was standing on the third step of a small ladder yesterday morning when he fell back and banged his chest on the rail of the stairs. He has had chest pain since but he couldn't sleep last night because he has become more breathless. Isabella grunts and turns away as he breathes deep into the mask. Examine him and…

⋯⟩ **390**

346 Ten minutes later you receive the request back from the x-ray department with a terse note telling you that 'imaging will not be performed in a clinical vacuum'. Suitably chastised, you go to examine the patient. **Deduct 1 point**.

⋯⟩ **361**

347 PFA of Lizzie Thurston

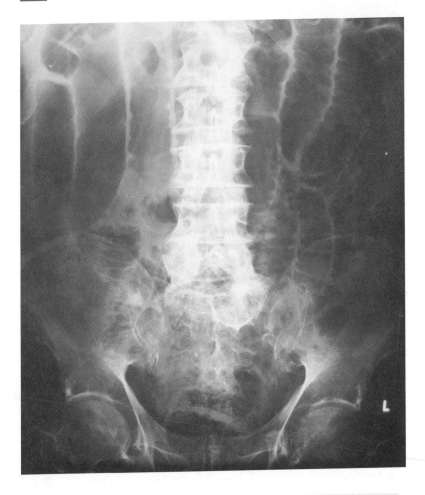

I. Nothing, observe for the moment ⋯⋗ **337**

II. Schedule theatre ⋯⋗ **403**

348 Eileen sighs as she tells you yes but he's a chest trauma. Embarrassed and weary, you go to look at the patient; **deduct 1 point**.

⋯⋗ **368**

349 No, with all things being equal you should attend to the small bowel obstruction first as she is potentially sicker; **deduct 1 point**.

⋯⋗ **419**

350 You ring Nicola to arrange theatre but Cahoon happens to be down in the anaesthetic office when you call. '*I can't leave you for a minute, Simpson. Forget it, I'll look after it,*' he tells you. **Deduct 1 point** and find a new patient.

⋯⋗ **401**

351 Al appreciates your honesty and appears a lot more settled. You leave him and his wife, wondering to yourself how they ever married, and go and check the slot one more time.

⋯⋗ **395**

352 You carefully mark the area around the dressing and admit for IV antibiotics. The following day Halsted is rounding and wants to know why on earth the wound wasn't opened to allow the collection to drain. Much to your embarrassment, he asks who was on call last night. Cahoon looks over, glaring at you as you step forward, and although there are 11 people around the bed, you can still hear Winston sniggering. Halsted looks at you and grins, slapping you on the back: '*Maybe not a surgeon, but a physician in the making,*' he says, walking away, and the mob laugh nervously. *Deduct 1 point* and go find your next patient.

⋯⋗ **334**

353 Yes, Lizzie appears to be dehydrated and is tachycardic. **Add 1 point**. You also decide to insert a catheter to monitor her urine output. Do you want to add in potassium?

   I. '*Yes* ⋯⋗ **340**

   II. *No* ⋯⋗ **412**

354 Yes, Lizzie appears to be dehydrated and is tachycardic. You also decide to insert a catheter to monitor her urine output. Do you want to add in potassium?

   I. *Yes* ⋯⋗ **369**

   II. *No* ⋯⋗ **400**

355 You haven't managed to pass this section but your score is a good one to build on. This section included a considerable amount of patient- and relative-based problems. These are not easy and often pose the most difficulty for us as there is no clear right or wrong and certainly no textbook answer. Repeat the section and aim to get above 14. Be clear on what the patient and their signs and symptoms are telling you. Remember, a doctor who cannot take a good history and a patient who cannot give one are in danger of giving and receiving bad treatment.

356 Al finds it difficult to give you a history with the mask on but he does manage to tell you that he was standing on the third step of a small ladder yesterday morning when he fell back and banged his chest on the stair rail. He has had chest pain since but he couldn't sleep last night because he has become more breathless. Isabella grunts and turns away. *'He's just trying to get out of having my sister over this week,'* she mutters.

Examine him and ⋯⟶ **390**

357 You tell him that you're really busy and you can't be wasting precious time on people who don't want to be helped, asking him if he realises just how many sick people are in the department. While you're waiting for an answer, the cubicle curtain is pulled back and you spin around to see Cahoon with a face like thunder. *'Simpson, get out of here,'* he growls. *'What are you playing at? Look, I'm tired and I really don't want to get into it now. I'll see this man,'* he says, taking the chart from you. *'Go and find somebody else, and never speak to a patient like that again or you're finished in this hospital.'* Chastised, you return to the slot and pull the next chart. **Deduct 1 point.**

⋯⟶ **401**

358 You explain to Al that he needs a chest drain so he's happy to go along with whatever you say. You prep him and insert a chest drain on the right side and it appears to be working properly. Al wants to know how long he'll have the chest drain in for and you explain that it's difficult to be exact as it will depend on his lung re-expanding. His wife grunts behind him: *'I guess he'll use this as an excuse to miss our holiday in 4 weeks'.* A little irritated, you ask Mrs Lopez to show a little more understanding as her husband has suffered a serious injury and is clearly not faking. Put out, she tells you that he probably did it on purpose. *'I have a flight in 4 weeks, doctor, do you think I'll be able to go?'* he asks. What will you tell him?

I. *I don't know but I'll ask somebody who does* ⋯⟶ **351**

II. *Yes* ⋯⟶ **329**

III. *No* ⋯⟶ **342**

359 You scored well and passed this section – good job. This section included a considerable amount of patient- and relative-based problems. These are not easy and often pose the most difficulty for us as there is no clear right or wrong and certainly no textbook answer. Always remember that your job is to improve your patient and, as James Bryce said, *'Medicine is the only profession that labours incessantly to destroy the reason for its own existence'.* Well done.

360 Yes, **add 1 point**. With all things being equal, a small bowel obstruction should be your priority.

⋯⟩ **419**

361 Lizzie gingerly lies back on the trolley for you. Her abdomen is distended and tympanic but is not tender. You can feel the staple line on rectal examination and it admits your digit with ease and no obvious obstruction. She has no hernia. What will you do next?

I. Give IV fluids ⋯⟩ **353**

II. Pass an NG tube ⋯⟩ **373**

III. Order radiology ⋯⟩ **396**

IV. Schedule theatre ⋯⟩ **403**

362 Eileen tells you that he is a 42-year-old man who sustained chest trauma yesterday and has had pain since. Glad you asked before looking like an idiot by telling her to get the medical team to see him, you go to see the patient.

⋯⟩ **368**

363 You decide not to send Johnny for counselling; **deduct 1 point**. Go to your next patient.

⋯⟩ **401**

364 OK, not a great score to finish with. Take a look at what went wrong. It may be that you made a bad decision early on in the book which resulted in you being sent home. Try the section again and this time think carefully before making a decision. There is no time limit to this book and just by being careful you will be able to increase your score.

365 You decide to treat the obstruction conservatively and Cahoon agrees. However, he asks you to get a PFA as he would like to have an idea of the level of obstruction. You do this and it shows a mid-ileal obstruction.

⋯⟩ **337**

366 Nicola puts the patient to sleep, and you pass a forceps per rectum and manage to grasp the corner of the rubber device. Very carefully, you bring it down through the rectum and deliver it out without causing any obvious damage. Do you want to perform a postremoval sigmoidoscopy?

I. Yes ⋯⟩ **338**

II. No ⋯⟩ **411**

367 You remove the four sutures that are holding the wound together and about 10 ml of pus oozes out as the skin opens. You gently wash out the wound, bringing relief to Elaine, leaving in a small wick. **Add 1 point.** What will you do now?

> I. *Clean the wound thoroughly and close it with some interrupted sutures* ⋯⟩ **393**

> II. *Leave it open and insert a wick* ⋯⟩ **413**

368 Walking over to examination room 3, you introduce yourself to Al Lopez. Al is sitting up and clearly a little breathless, taking shallow short breaths. His wife is sitting beside him looking in the other direction. With difficulty Al tells you that he is 42 years old. You glance at the monitor and his oxygen saturations are 91%. What do you want to do next?

> I. *Give oxygen through a face mask and take a history from his wife* ⋯⟩ **345**

> II. *Give oxygen through a facemask and take a history from Al* ⋯⟩ **356**

> III. *Give oxygen through nasal prongs and take a history from Al* ⋯⟩ **335**

> IV. *Quickly take the history first before giving oxygen* ⋯⟩ **397**

369 You add potassium to her fluids. **Add 1 point.** What will you do next?

> I. *Order radiology* ⋯⟩ **376**

> II. *Organise theatre* ⋯⟩ **403**

> III. *Nothing, observe for the moment* ⋯⟩ **365**

370 You explain fully to Al that he has a pneumothorax and will require a chest drain. He is happy to do whatever is necessary. You prep him and insert a chest drain into his left side. Two hours later his O_2 sats are continuing to fall and you review him with Cahoon. '*The chest drain is oscillating,*' he observes, '*I'm not sure why he's still dropping his sats, unless he has another pneumothorax on the right. Let's see his x-ray,*' he says, pulling out the film. '*Yes, see this Simpson, quite a large one on the right . . . hang on, he's got no pneumothorax on the left.*' The full realisation of what has happened hits both you and him simultaneously. Your days in Pilgrims are over and you'll be lucky if that's the worst that happens.

371 You mark the area and prescribe oral antibiotics. Two days later you review Elaine and her cellulitis has settled completely, with her wound healing nicely. **Add 1 point** and go to your next patient.

> ⋯⟩ **334**

372 Annabel is horrified and refuses to believe you, telling you that she is on her way to the hospital now and wants to see you and her husband. She puts the phone down on you; **deduct 1 point**. She arrives 2 hours later and causes a scene in the reception area of the hospital with Cahoon. One week later, Halsted receives a letter of complaint from Johnny Wassan for breach of confidentiality. What a disaster.

Although Johnny's behaviour may not be to your taste, will you encourage him to attend counselling for potential infectious diseases?

> *I. Yes* ⋯⟩ **408**

> *II. No, it is the patient's own personal business* ⋯⟩ **363**

373 Do you want to pass a:

> *I. Wide-bore tube* ⋯⟩ **328**

> *II. Narrow-bore tube* ⋯⟩ **388**

374 Chest X-ray of Al Lopez. **Add 1 point**. What will you do next?

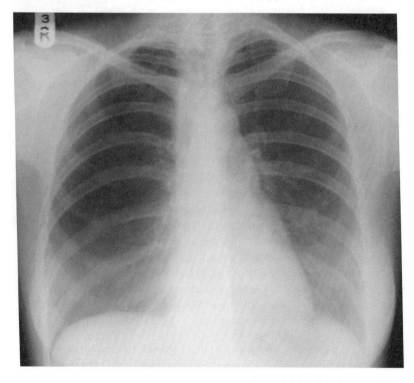

I. Allow home on analgesia ⸺⫸ 428

II. Admit and observe overnight ⸺⫸ 389

III. Insert a chest drain ⸺⫸ 394

375 You exaggerate the rate of wound infections to try and placate her and she seems to believe you. However, 2 weeks later Halsted gets a legal letter complaining that not only did she suffer a postoperative complication but that the doctors and hospital tried to cover it up by lying to her. Halsted is furious and the last you see of him is as he thunders down the corridor looking for the *'idiot who was on call that night'*. Knowing that this isn't going to be pleasant, you keep your head down. **Deduct 1 point**. Right now, you need to decide what to do next with Elaine. Will you:

I. Mark the area and allow home on oral antibiotics and review in your clinic in 2 days ⸺⫸ 371

II. Mark the area and admit for IV antibiotics ⸺⫸ 402

376 What would you like to order?

I. PFA ⸺⫸ 347

II. CT abdomen ⸺⫸ 339

377 To get a better idea of what's going on, you gently begin to palpate his abdomen. Placing your hand over his umbilicus, you feel a slow gentle buzzing. Baffled, it takes you a few seconds to realise what has happened.

⸺⫸ **424**

378 You carefully mark the area around the dressing and allow home on antibiotics. Two days later Elaine represents to Pilgrims with pus oozing from her wound. Winston deftly snips the sutures and opens the wound, allowing it to drain. He cleans the wound and photographs it, using the pictures to supplement his next teaching presentation, relishing telling the audience about the wound collection that was missed. **Deduct 1 point** and go find your next patient.

⸺⫸ **334**

379 Immediately you grab a 14 gauge cannula and, getting Al to sit back, you drive it into the second intercostal space on the right-hand side. Al roars as the cannula goes in and his wife starts screaming hysterically. One of the emergency doctors is passing and runs in when she hears the commotion. *'What the hell is going on in here?'* she demands. You try to explain that this man has a tension pneumothorax and you've just saved his life. She looks at you incredulously. *'He walked in from the waiting room and* *has been sitting on this trolley for the last 30 minutes – he does not have a tension pneumothorax.'* Margaret tries to console Isabella who is screaming hysterically. '*He tried to kill my husband*,' she yells. The emergency doctor tells you to leave and 10 minutes later Cahoon finds you in the coffee room, '*What the hell were you thinking, Simpson?*' he asks but before you can answer, he tells you to get your stuff and get out, your days in Pilgrims are over.

380 Before you have a chance to get the chest drain in, Margaret has contacted Cahoon and he asks for you on the phone. '*What on earth are you doing, Simpson? I don't care who you think you are, I want that pneumothorax confirmed before you start sticking tubes into people. In fact, forget it, I'll do it myself. Go look for another patient.*'

→ **395**

381 Calculate your scores from section 3.

I. *If you scored a negative figure* → **364**

II. *If you scored between 1 and 14* → **355**

III. *If you scored between 15 and 21* → **359**

IV. *If you scored >22* → **398**

382 You also decide to insert a catheter to monitor her urine output. Do you want to add in potassium?

I. *Yes* → **369**

II. *No* → **400**

383 You ring Cahoon and tell him your plans. He tells you to hang on as it might be possible to get it out without a laparotomy. **Deduct 1 point**.

→ **366**

384 Yes, more information always helps. **Add 1 point**. The 27-year-old lady has had periumbilical pain and vomiting for 24 hours. She has a BP of 118/67 and a pulse of 112 and has a normal temperature. The 21-year-old lady has noticed some redness and tenderness around her wound site from an open appendectomy 6 days ago. Her BP is 122/73, pulse 68 and she has a normal temperature. Who will you review first?

I. *The 27 year old* → **360**

II. *The 21 year old* → **349**

385 Elaine thanks you for your honesty, and 2 weeks later Halsted gets a legal letter stating that had he been a more skilled surgeon, Ms Cardosa would not have suffered a wound infection. Halsted is furious, swearing and shouting about jumped-up idiot lawyers who know nothing about surgery. **Deduct 1 point**. When this happens, you keep your head down. Right now, you need to decide what to do next with Elaine. Will you:

> *I. Mark the area and allow home on oral antibiotics and review in your clinic in 2 days* ⸱⸱⸳ **371**
>
> *II. Mark the area and admit for IV antibiotics* ⸱⸱⸳ **402**

386 You tell Elaine the truth and she appreciates it as you explain that infections do happen in about 23% of complicated appendectomies. Happy with your explanation, she wants to know if she can go home. **Add 1 point**. Will you:

> *I. Mark the area and allow home on oral antibiotics and review in your clinic in 2 days* ⸱⸱⸳ **371**
>
> *II. Mark the area and admit for IV antibiotics* ⸱⸱⸳ **402**

387 You lie to Annabel and she seems to believe you although she sounds suspicious; **deduct 1 point** for lying. Although Johnny's behaviour may not be to your taste, will you encourage him to attend counselling for potential infectious diseases?

> *I. Yes* ⸱⸱⸳ **408**
>
> *II. No, it is the patient's own personal business* ⸱⸱⸳ **363**

388 Joy is the nurse helping you and you ask her where you would find a narrow-bore nasogastric tube. She points over to the press but asks if maybe you mean a wide bore as you need it for drainage rather than feeding? Realising your mistake, you quickly recover: *'Yes, did I say narrow bore? Sorry! It's been a long night'*. **Deduct 1 point**. You carefully pass the tube and immediately aspirate 2300 ml from Lizzie's stomach; instantly she feels more comfortable. What will you do next?

> *I. Give IV fluids* ⸱⸱⸳ **354**
>
> *II. Order radiology* ⸱⸱⸳ **414**
>
> *III. Schedule theatre* ⸱⸱⸳ **403**

389 Fortunately Cahoon does a ward round an hour later and reviews Al, who by now is beginning to tire from his increased respiratory rate. *'What are you doing, Simpson? This guy is hypoxic, tachypneic and has a large traumatic pneumothorax, he clearly needs a chest drain.'* Winston just loves these ward rounds. **Deduct 1 point**. Right now, you leave Al in the emergency department and return to check the slot one more time.

⋯⟩ **395**

390 Al's pulse is 105, BP 156/100, respiratory rate 22 and his ABG can be found in the Investigations at the end of this section. The air entry over his right lung is decreased and his trachea is in the midline. What will you do next?

> I. Immediately stick a wide-bore cannula in the second intercostal space on the right side ⋯⟩ **379**

> II. Get a chest x-ray ⋯⟩ **374**

> III. Put in a chest drain ⋯⟩ **427**

391 You back down and order the chest film you should have already done. **Deduct 1 point**.

⋯⟩ **394**

392 Joy is the nurse helping you and you ask her where you would find a narrow-bore nasogastric tube. She points over to the press but asks if maybe you mean a wide bore as you need it for drainage rather than feeding? Realising your mistake, you quickly recover: *'Yes, did I say narrow bore? Sorry! It's been a long night'*. **Deduct 1 point**. You carefully pass the tube and immediately aspirate 2300 ml from Lizzie's stomach; instantly she feels more comfortable. What will you do next?

> I. Nothing, observe for the moment ⋯⟩ **365**

> II. Order radiology ⋯⟩ **376**

> III. Schedule theatre ⋯⟩ **403**

393 You close the wound but unfortunately she develops another collection and this needs to be opened again 2 days from now. **Deduct 1 point**. However, right now, Elaine feels much improved but she does seem a little suspicious, asking *'Is this a complication of the surgeon not being able to take my appendix out using the keyhole technique?'*. What will you tell her?

> I. Yes, had the surgeon had more skill and been able to take the appendix out laparoscopically, this would not have happened ⋯⟩ **385**

> II. No, wound infections occur in laparoscopic appendectomies as much as open appendectomies ⋯⟩ **405**

> III. No, in complicated appendectomies wound infections occur in 23% of cases ⋯⟩ **386**

394 Recognising the pneumothorax and given that Al is hypoxic and symptomatic, you decide to put in a chest drain. **Add 1 point.** Which side will you put it in?

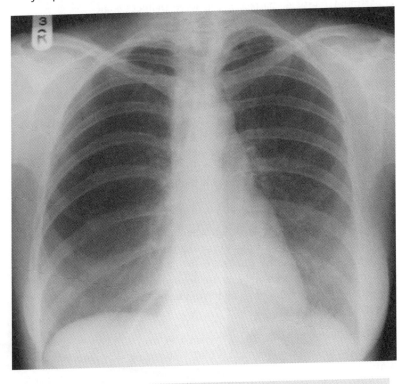

I. Right ⋯⟶ **358**

II. Left ⋯⟶ **370**

395 You return to the slot, the need for sleep overwhelming you now, and your heart sinks when you see another chart. Just as you reach for it, Winston grabs the chart and walks off. *'Let the real doctors take over now, Simpson, it's 8.10'*, he says. Far too tired to argue and relieved that your first night on call is finally done, you grab a quick shower. Halsted and Cahoon are just finishing a meeting and your ward round has been mercifully delayed. Just enough time now to get changed and feel half human again. Remember, no matter how bad it gets and no matter how busy it is, they can't stop the clock. Well done.

⋯⟶ **381**

396 You are just filling out a request when Joy observes that Lizzie appears quite dry and is still tachycardic, asking if you think it might be a good idea to give her some fluid before sending her down to the x-ray department. A little embarrassed, you agree. **Deduct 1 point**.

⋯⟩ 382

397 Breathlessly, he tells you that yesterday morning he was standing on the third step of a small ladder when he fell back and banged his chest on the rail of the stairs. He has had chest pain since but he couldn't sleep last night because he has become more breathless. Isabella grunts and turns away, muttering *'He just wants to get out of having my sister over this weekend'*. Al goes on to tell you that he has smoked about 20 cigarettes a day for the past 25 years but does not have any other medical problems. At this stage, Eileen comes in and sees that Al's oxygen saturations are just 88% and puts a face mask. on him. **Deduct 1 point** and examine him.

⋯⟩ 390

398 A perfect score. This is, without needing to say it, a very difficult task. This section included a considerable amount of patient- and relative-based problems. These are not easy to deal with and you have shown an ability to read between the lines and exercise good judgement in interpersonal matters along with a thorough understanding of the scientific aspects of patient care. Well done.

399 You push him harder to try to elicit a history but he is very slow to engage and lies back, pulling up his shirt. Not getting anywhere, you exam him.

⋯⟩ 377

400 You give her fluids without potassium. **Deduct 1 point**. What will you do next?

   I. Order radiology ⋯⟩ **376**

   II. Organise theatre ⋯⟩ **403**

   III. Nothing, observe for the moment ⋯⟩ **365**

401 Deftly avoiding a drunk who is standing in the middle of the department shouting, you make your way back to the slot. There are two patients to be seen. The first is a 27-year-old lady who has been triaged as a possible small bowel obstruction, and the second is a 21-year-old lady who has a possible wound infection after an open appendectomy. What will you do next?

402 You admit Elaine overnight and she is seen on the ward round in the morning. Halsted is surprised to see her back but happy she has been looked after. He switches her IV antibiotics to oral antibiotics and allows her home. Go to see your next patient.

⋯⟩ **334**

403 You ring Nicola and tell her that you have a bowel obstruction that needs to go to theatre. Nicola cancels an orthopaedic case she is about to start in order to give priority to your case. You tell Cahoon, who tells you to hold off until he has seen the patient. Ten minutes later, he rings you back to say that she's probably an adhesive obstruction and you should drain with the NG tube, replace her fluids and electrolytes, monitor her urine output and watch her overnight. Embarrassed, you tell him about booking theatre. *'Not a great call, Simpson. Tell you what, I'll ring Nicola and let her know, but I'd stay away from her until she calms down.'* Sheepishly, you go to see the patient with the wound infection. **Deduct 1 point**.

⋯⟩ **407**

404 You ring Cahoon to tell him what you're planning and he tells you to get a PFA first to find the position of the device.

⋯⟩ **331**

405 You lie and tell her that it would not have made a difference. She appears to believe you but 2 weeks later Halsted gets a legal letter complaining that not only did she suffer a postoperative complication but that the doctors and hospital tried to cover it up by lying to her. Halsted is furious and the last you see of him is as he thunders down the corridor looking for the *'idiot who was on call that night'*. Knowing that this isn't going to be pleasant, you keep your head down. **Deduct 1 point**. Right now, you need to decide what to do next with Elaine. Will you:

I. Mark the area and allow home on oral antibiotics and review in your clinic in 2 days ⋯⟩ **371**

II. Mark the area and admit for IV antibiotics ⋯⟩ **402**

406 PFA of Lizzie Thurston.

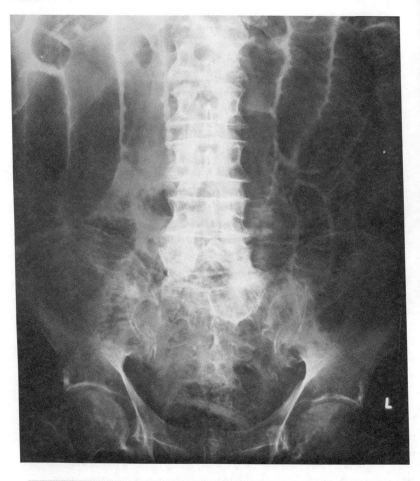

I. Nothing, observe for the moment ⋯⟩ **337**

II. Schedule theatre ⋯⟩ **403**

407 You spend 5 minutes trying to track down your next patient, Elaine Cardosa, and finally find that she's been moved to a new cubicle. You introduce yourself to the young lady sitting on the trolley. Seven days ago, she had a laparoscopic appendectomy which was converted to an open procedure when it was found that her appendix was quite stuck and difficult to remove. She stayed in hospital for 2 days and was discharged. For the last 36 hours she has had pain and redness around the site but no other systemic features. Exam her.

⋯⟩ **410**

408 Good decision; **add 1 point**. Johnny's behaviour poses a high risk to himself and his wife, who clearly is not fully aware. He should be counselled on testing for sexually transmitted infectious diseases. Go to your next patient.

⋯⟩ **401**

409 **Add 1 point**. You ask him when the pain began and he mutters that it started about 4 hours ago. You ask him whether he has had any other symptoms such as nausea or vomiting but he shakes his head. You quickly realise that you are not getting very far. He tells you that he doesn't want anybody to know that he is here. What would you like to do next?

I. Examine him ⋯⟩ **377**

II. Tell him that you're really busy and that unless he tells you what's wrong, you'll go and see somebody else ⋯⟩ **357**

410 Ubeki steps in while you exam Elaine. Her abdomen is flat and there is a dressing over the incision site. There is erythema extending around the edges of the dressing. She is quite tender over the dressing but has no other tenderness in her abdomen. What will you do next?

I. Take down the dressing ⋯⟩ **426**

II. Leave the dressing undisturbed, mark the area and admit her for IV antibiotics ⋯⟩ **352**

III. Don't disturb the dressing, mark the area and allow her home with oral antibiotics ⋯⟩ **378**

411 You decide not to perform a postremoval sigmoidoscopy. **Deduct 1 point**.

⋯⟩ **425**

412 You give her fluids without potassium. **Deduct 1 point**. Her abdomen is distended and tympanic but not tender. You can feel the staple line on rectal examination and it admits your digit with ease and no obvious stricture. She has no hernia. What will you do next?

I. Order radiology ⋯⟩ **376**

II. Pass an NG tube ⋯⟩ **418**

III. Organise theatre ⋯⟩ **403**

IV. Nothing, observe for the moment ⋯⟩ **333**

413 You leave the wound open to heal by secondary intention so as not to trap bacteria within the wound. Right now, Elaine feels much improved but

Section 3

she seems a little suspicious, asking *'Is this a complication of the surgeon not being able to take my appendix out using the keyhole technique?'*. What will you tell her?

> I. *Yes, had the surgeon had more skill and been able to take the appendix out laparoscopically, this would not have happened* ⋯⟩ **385**

> II. *No, wound infections occur in laparoscopic appendectomies as much as open appendectomies* ⋯⟩ **405**

> III. *No, in complicated appendectomies wound infections occur in 23% of cases* ⋯⟩ **386**

414 You are just filling out a request when Joy observes that Lizzie appears quite dry and is still tachycardic, asking if you think it might be a good idea to give her some fluid before sending her down to the x-ray department. A little embarrassed, you agree. **Deduct 1 point**.

⋯⟩ **376**

415 You call Nicola and bring the patient down to theatre for an EUA. **Add 1 point**.

⋯⟩ **366**

416 You tell her that it would be safer to cancel and reschedule it. Lizzie becomes upset and begins to panic: *'The flowers, the church, the cake ...'* Margaret, who was outside, steps in and tries to calm her, telling her that it's early yet and it may settle in time, explaining that the doctors will have a far better idea over the next 24 hours as to what will happen. *'Doctor, don't you have another patient to see?'* Margaret asks, glaring at you. Sheepishly, you slip out from behind the curtain and go to see your lady with the wound infection. **Deduct 1 point**.

⋯⟩ **407**

417 Well handled. You have not lied, but neither have you broken your patient's confidence. **Add 1 point**. Although Johnny's behaviour may not be to your taste, will you encourage him to attend counselling for potential infectious diseases?

> I. *Yes* ⋯⟩ **408**

> II. *No, it is the patient's own personal business* ⋯⟩ **363**

418 Do you want to pass a:

> I. *Wide bore tube* ⋯⟩ **330**

> II. *Narrow bore tube* ⋯⟩ **392**

419 Behind the curtain, you find Lizzie Thurston, a 27-year-old lady who had a panproctocolectomy and ileoanal pouch 4 years ago for ulcerative colitis. She made a good recovery and has been trouble free since. She developed crampy pain around her umbilicus with associated vomiting 24 hours ago and has not passed any bowel motion or flatus since. She has been crying and tells you that she is due to be married in 6 days' time. She is otherwise comfortable at the moment and you complete your history with little else remarkable. Her bloods can be found in the Investigations at the end of this section. What will you do next?

> *I. Examine her* ⋯⟩ **423**
>
> *II. Give IV fluids* ⋯⟩ **353**
>
> *III. Order a PFA* ⋯⟩ **336**

420 You put down on the form that she has a distended abdomen and mild generalised tenderness. Fifteen minutes later, Cahoon comes looking for you. *'Simpson, you've stepped over the line here, nobody has examined this patient. This lady has a ileostomy and an incarcerated parastomal hernia and is locally peritonitic. I think it's ischaemic.'* You feel your stomach drop at being caught, silently cursing the woman for not mentioning the stoma to you. You don't even try to make an excuse. *'It's one thing you not knowing something, Simpson, but it's downright dangerous having a liar on the service. Give me your bleep and make an appointment to see Halsted in the morning.'* He takes your bleep and you gather your bag, not noticing the bitter cold air outside as the doors slide behind you.

421 You tell her not to do anything hasty at the moment as you'll have a far better idea over the next 24 hours as to whether or not this is going to settle without an operation. She seems to accept this and you promise to let her know the minute anything changes. **Add 1 point**.

⋯⟩ **407**

422 You are about to discharge when Margaret becomes concerned and rings Cahoon. *'Put Simpson on the phone to me,'* he tells her. *'What are you doing, Simpson? I can't take this any more, you're simply reckless. Leave him and I'll see him and sort him out.'* Before you can say anything in reply, the phone is put down and you sheepishly go back to the slot for the next patient. **Deduct 1 point**.

⋯⟩ **401**

423 Lizzie gingerly lies back on the trolley for you. Her abdomen is distended and tympanic but not tender. You can feel the staple line on rectal examination and it admits your digit with ease and no obvious stricture. She has no hernia. **Add 1 point**. What will you do next?

424 You ask him how long the vibrator has been in his rectum and he tells you about 36 hours. He was a paying customer with a male escort service in town and they both tried getting it out but just managed to push it further in. The rest of his abdomen is soft and non-tender and on examining his rectum, there is no sign of the device. You try to figure out what you're going to do when he asks you '*How long will it keep buzzing, doctor?*'. Thinking that it really depends on what type of batteries he uses, you decide not to ask and tell him that you don't know but you'll have to figure out a way of removing it. You perform a rectal examination but cannot feel or see the vibrator. What will you do next?

I. *Organise an examination under anaesthesia* ⋯⟩ **404**

II. *Organise theatre for a colectomy* ⋯⟩ **350**

III. *Order a PFA* ⋯⟩ **343**

IV. *Order a CT* ⋯⟩ **429**

425 Nicola reverses the anaesthetic and Johnny is brought out to the recovery room. Just as you're finishing up, the theatre nurse hands you the phone and tells you that it's Annabel Wassan, the patient's wife. She was worried when he had not contacted her and has been ringing around the city. When she heard he was in Pilgrims Hospital and that he was undergoing emergency surgery, she became frightened and wants to know how her husband is and what happened to him. What do you want to tell her?

I. *The truth* ⋯⟩ **372**

II. *That he had a fall and you had to examine him to make sure he was all right, but he'll be fine and should be discharged tomorrow* ⋯⟩ **387**

III. *That you don't like discussing details over the phone, but that her husband is in no danger and should be discharged tomorrow, and you will ask him to ring her later when he is fully awake* ⋯⟩ **417**

426 Naturally you want to look at the wound; **add 1 point**. Elaine winces as you carefully take off the dressing. The dressing is stained with amber pus and the wound is swollen and leaking pus from between the sutures. It is red around the wound, and Elaine's tenderness is limited to only the wound itself. What will you do next?

I. Take out the sutures ⋯⇢ **367**

II. Mark the area and admit her for IV antibiotics ⋯⇢ **352**

III. Mark the area and allow her home with oral antibiotics ⋯⇢ **378**

427 You prep for a chest drain. Margaret asks if you're going to get a chest x-ray first. Will you:

I. Tell her it's a clinical decision ⋯⇢ **380**

II. Get a chest x-ray ⋯⇢ **391**

428 You prescribe strong analgesia for Al and allow him home. However, the large pneumothorax combined with the respiratory depression caused by him taking an excess of codeine in an attempt to control the pain results in him returning to the department 8 hours later in full respiratory arrest. By the time he reaches hospital, he has been down for about an hour and it is not possible to resuscitate him. You happen to be on a ward round passing through the emergency department when his wife sees you and lunges at you, screaming that you killed her husband. Security pull her away from you but the resulting investigation shows that you misdiagnosed a serious injury and your treatment was negligent. You will have to face a fitness to practise enquiry but in the meantime your career at Pilgrims is over.

429 You ring Ruth and ask her to perform a CT scan to locate the device. Ruth suggests that plain film of his abdomen may show you as easily where it is and if that doesn't clarify it then she will do a CT scan.

⋯⇢ **331**

PERSPECTIVES

Case perspectives: Johnny Wasson

THERAPEUTIC PERSPECTIVES

1 Difficult history taking

- There are several reasons why healthcare professionals fail to take a sexual history, including fear of offending the patient, no relevance and a perceived lack of training.[1,2]
- Open-ended questions and explaining why such questions are necessary[3] are both strategies to overcome these issues.

JOHNNY AND HISTORY TAKING

Johnny is a difficult historian who is clearly reluctant to talk about what has happened. Initially, you are not given an indication that this may be a sexual problem. Additionally, as he has insisted on seeing the surgeon first, one can postulate that this is not the first time that something like this has happened and he 'knows the procedure'. The best you can do in such situations is to stick to your training of trying to take a history as well as possible, and in as sensitive and professional a manner as possible.

2 Retained rectal foreign bodies

- The real incidence is unknown as most patients will present only with perforations or who are unable or unwilling to remove the foreign body.[4,5]
- Patients are more likely to present with a complaint of a retained foreign body rather than pain or symptoms.[4]
- Patients usually have tried to remove the foreign body prior to presentation.[6]
- When there is no need for urgent surgical intervention, a trial period of waiting for the object to pass may be successful, even with objects in the sigmoid (45%).[4]
- Following this, a bedside extraction through digital manipulation may be successful in up to 75% of cases.[4]
- When these approaches fail, an examination under anaesthesia is the most common surgical approach to removal, with a laparotomy only considered for those with signs of peritonitis or in whom the above attempts have failed.[4]
- All published treatment strategies recommend performing a postremoval sigmoidoscopy[4] in order to rule out significant rectal and colonic trauma.

JOHNNY AND THE RETAINED FOREIGN BODY

The vibrator has not passed in nearly 48 hours and your attempts at localising it through a rectal examination have failed. You are now faced with deciding the next step. Johnny is not systemically unwell and so an EUA would be the next appropriate step. There are many approaches, including using a soft balloon catheter or rigid sigmoidoscopy, but in this case you would have managed to use a soft-tipped grasper to safely remove it. Failing to attempt an EUA first before proceeding to laparotomy would have resulted in you losing marks, as would failing to do a postremoval sigmoidoscopy.

3 Confidentiality

- Privacy is a principle derived from autonomy and covers a patient's intimacy, honour and image. It is the healthcare professional's duty to protect this.[7]
- In the case where there is a threat to another person's life, such as HIV infection, confidentiality may be breached to inform the patient's spouse or other 'at risk' individuals.[8]

JOHNNY AND CONFIDENTIALITY

Currently you do not know if Johnny is a threat to his wife's life, as you are not aware of his infection status. However, clearly he is potentially endangering her with high-risk sexual behaviour. Certainly, over the telephone in a busy theatre is not the way in which to explore this further. Johnny should be counselled regarding testing for sexually transmitted diseases. If you failed to do this, you were docked points. Attempts to encourage the patient to tell their spouse or other at-risk individual should be exhausted before breaking a patient's confidence, but another individual should not be allowed to be put at risk.

COMMUNICATION PERSPECTIVES

Annabel's perspective

- Annabel is under the impression that her husband is away on business.
- Johnny has travelled 100 miles to conceal his behaviour.
- Annabel has not heard from him and rings around the hospitals.

SIMPSON AND ANNABEL

Obviously, what is happening to Annabel is wrong and apart from the betrayal and hurt she will inevitably feel, Johnny is potentially putting her at risk of sexually transmitted diseases. Clearly, this is something you need to get involved in and not ignore. However, discussing this on a telephone is obviously inappropriate. Also, lying to Annabel, who has already been lied to by the person she loves, is not appropriate. This is a difficult position to be in and calls for tact and understanding. Explaining that you cannot go into the details over the phone but reassuring her that Johnny is safe is the best strategy. Obviously, there are issues to be discussed but this should be done in a more controlled and sensitive manner.

Johnny's perspective

- Johnny is concealing his behaviour from his wife; he is clearly unsatisfied with elements of his life.
- He has not been honest with his wife regarding his sexual tendencies and this potentially puts her at risk.
- He is embarrassed by what has happened and is reluctant to discuss it, making him a difficult historian.
- He has asked for the surgeon, which may be a clue that this is not the first time it has happened.
- Coming to hospital is not going to be his first choice and so you can imagine that he has tried to remove the object himself.

SIMPSON AND JOHNNY

You are in a difficult position, but Johnny has come looking for help and he is your patient. Regardless of your opinion, he deserves your professionalism and help. This may be an opportunity for a healthcare professional to become involved and save both Johnny and those around him from potential danger, and so the opportunity should not be lost. In a situation like this, there is inevitable 'interest' in the case from your colleagues. However, you should try to remember that although many may find it humorous, it is a tragic and potentially dangerous situation for the people involved, who may ultimately come to learn that they are infected with a serious disease or it may signal the end to their marriage.

What happened to Johnny?

Johnny agreed to be tested for sexually transmitted diseases and fortunately tested negative. He had been a regular customer of male prostitutes in the city for over a year and was unhappy in the sexual element of his marriage. He was afraid to split from his wife as he wanted to conceal his sexual preferences, especially from his children. In the end, he and his wife decided to give their marriage another try. To date, they are still together.

Section 3

REFERENCE LIST

1. Risen CB. A guide to taking a sexual history. Psychiatr Clin North Am 1995;18(1):39–53.

2. Merrill JM, Laux LF, Thornby JI. Why doctors have difficulty with sex histories. South Med J 1990;83(6):613–617.

3. Longworth JC. Sexual assessment and counseling in primary care. Nurse Pract Forum 1997;8(4):166–171.

4. Lake JP, Essani R, Petrone P, Kaiser AM, Asensio J, Beart RW Jr. Management of retained colorectal foreign bodies: predictors of operative intervention. Dis Colon Rectum 2004;47(10):1694–1698.

5. Barone JE, Sohn N, Nealon TF Jr. Perforations and foreign bodies of the rectum: report of 28 cases. Ann Surg 1976;184(5):601–604.

6. Crass RA, Tranbaugh RF, Kudsk KA, Trunkey DD. Colorectal foreign bodies and perforation. Am J Surg 1981;142(1):85–88.

7. Heikkinen AM, Wickstrom GJ, Leino-Kilpi H. Privacy in occupational health practice: promoting and impeding factors. Scand J Public Health 2007; 35(2):116–124.

8. Sirinskiene A, Juskevicius J, Naberkovas A. Confidentiality and duty to warn the third parties in HIV/AIDS context. Med Etika Bioet 2005; 12(1):2–7.

Case perspectives: Lizzie Thurston

THERAPEUTIC PERSPECTIVES

1 Adhesions

- One study attempted to quantify the problem of adhesions and found that of 210 patients undergoing a laparotomy who had had previous surgery, 93% had adhesions.[1]
- Adhesions are less common after transverse incisions than midline incisions.[2]
- Bleeding, infection and visceral injury increase the incidence of adhesions, while laparoscopy appears to decrease the incidence.[3–5]
- In a small bowel obstruction several litres of crystalloid are often required for resuscitation along with potassium supplementation. Patients with a long history often present with an alkalosis and hypokalaemia due to hydrogen ion loss and renal compensation.[6]
- Decompression with a nasogastric tube will reduce vomiting, decompress the bowel and reduce the risk of aspiration.[6]

LIZZIE AND ADHESIONS

Adhesions are the most common cause of small bowel obstruction and the likely reason for Lizzie's presentation. She needs resuscitation with electrolyte replacement, gastric decompression and analgesia. Failure to follow these steps will result in you being deducted points.

2 When to operate

- There are no absolute criteria for when to operate on a patient with adhesional small bowel obstruction.[7]
- In patients with multiple laparotomies and no signs of strangulation, it is often prudent to monitor past 24–48 hours with the use of parenteral feeding where necessary. Any signs of strangulation such as tenderness, pyrexia or tachycardia should warrant surgical exploration.[6]
- Successful laparoscopic management of adhesional small bowel obstruction has been reported but access is often difficult and it requires a skilled laparoscopic surgeon.[7]
- Laparoscopy has also found a role in those patients managed conservatively and then brought back for elective intervention.[8]

LIZZIE AND OPERATING

Lizzie has a short history and certainly warrants an attempt at conservative management. If this fails, surgical exploration will be necessary but starting with such an approach would have cost you points.

COMMUNICATION PERSPECTIVES

Lizzie's perspective

- Lizzie is getting married in 6 days time.
- Obviously she is distraught at the thought of having to cancel her wedding.
- It is possible that a small bowel obstruction will have settled by this time.

SIMPSON AND LIZZIE

Clearly, there is a chance that Lizzie can still make her wedding in 6 days time. Either way, there is nothing she can do about it at 6am, and the next few hours will provide considerably more prognostic information. This is an opportunity to be calm and try to explain that the next 24 hours will let you know with far more certainty. Panicking Lizzie by telling her to cancel her wedding resulted in you being deducted points.

Margaret's perspective

- Margaret does not want to see her patient upset.
- She responds to your lack of sensitivity by doing what you should have done – that is, to try to calm Lizzie and explain that the next 24 hours will tell a lot.
- Margaret displays her impatience with you by reminding you that there are other patients to see.

SIMPSON AND MARGRET

If you told Lizzie to cancel her wedding, you have made an error by panicking her. Fortunately, Margaret has recovered the situation. Although embarrassing, her put-down is a small price to pay for your patient's comfort.

What happened to Lizzie?

Lizzie's small bowel obstruction settled very quickly without surgical intervention. She resumed diet late the following day and was discharged after 48 hours. She got married as planned 3 days after discharge, sending the department a bouquet of flowers on her wedding day. At the time of writing, she has not re-presented.

REFERENCE LIST

1. Menzies D, Ellis H. Intestinal obstruction from adhesions – how big is the problem? Ann R Coll Surg Engl 1990;72(1):60–63.

2. Brill AI, Nezhat F, Nezhat CH, Nezhat C. The incidence of adhesions after prior laparotomy: a laparoscopic appraisal. Obstet Gynecol 1995;85(2):269–272.

3. Wallwiener D, Meyer A, Bastert G. Adhesion formation of the parietal and visceral peritoneum: an explanation for the controversy on the use of autologous and alloplastic barriers? Fertil Steril 1998;69(1):132–137.

4. Gadallah MF, Torres-Rivera C, Ramdeen G, Myrick S, Habashi S, Andrews G. Relationship between intraperitoneal bleeding, adhesions, and peritoneal dialysis catheter failure: a method of prevention. Adv Perit Dial 2001;17:127–129.

5. Gamal EM, Metzger P, Szabo G, et al. The influence of intraoperative complications on adhesion formation during laparoscopic and conventional cholecystectomy in an animal model. Surg Endosc 2001;15(8):873–877.

6. Paterson-Brown S. *Core Topics in General and Emergency Surgery*, 3rd edn. Edinburgh: Elsevier, 2006.

7. Moran BJ. Adhesion-related small bowel obstruction. Colorectal Dis 2007;9(Suppl 2):39–44.

8. Tsumura H, Ichikawa T, Murakami Y, Sueda T. Laparoscopic adhesiolysis for recurrent postoperative small bowel obstruction. Hepatogastroenterology 2004;51(58):1058–1061.

Case perspectives: Elaine Cardosa

THERAPEUTIC PERSPECTIVES

1 Examining and treating the wound infection

- The classic signs of infection are rubor (redness), calor (heat), dolor (pain) and tumor (swelling).[1]
- Classic management of a wound infection includes drainage of any collection or pus by removing some of the sutures and gently probing the wound to break down the loculations. The wound is dressed regularly and not resutured, instead being allowed to heal by secondary intention.[2]
- If there is evidence of cellulitis, antibiotics should be given.[2]

Simpson and treatment of wound infection

Obviously it is impossible to assess the signs of infection without exposing the wound fully, so if you failed to do this you were deducted points. The classic treatment of a wound infection requires drainage of infected material and the prevention of further collections by not closing the wound. The presence of cellulitis requires treatment with antibiotics. Failure to follow these principles resulted in you losing marks. It is interesting that these instinctive principles have not been subjected to any large and reliable randomised clinical trials, presumably because of the intuitive nature of this approach.

2 Wound infections in laparoscopic surgery

- Wound infections have been shown to be half as likely after laparoscopic appendectomy as opposed to open appendectomy but initially it was suggested that laparoscopic appendectomy may increase the rate of intra-abdominal collections.[3]
- Laparoscopic appendectomy has also been shown to reduce the length of hospital stay from 2.9 to 2.1 days.[4]
- The hospital cost associated with laparoscopy is higher than with open surgery but the costs outside the hospital, including a return to normal activities, are less, with laparoscopy resulting in an overall society saving especially with actively employed patients.[5,6]
- In complicated appendicitis the rate of infection is higher than in uncomplicated pathology (23%).[7]
- A Cochrane review has concluded that laparoscopic appendectomy is recommended over open surgery unless laparoscopy is contraindicated or not feasible.[3]

SIMPSON AND WOUND INFECTIONS

Elaine had a difficult appendectomy as demonstrated by the fact that it was started laparoscopically and had to be converted to open. While overall laparoscopic appendectomy results in a reduced rate of wound infections, laparoscopy was not feasible in this case. As you were not present at the original surgery and could not appreciate the difficulties, telling Elaine that the surgeon was not skilled enough and that this was responsible for her infection is inappropriate and you were deducted points for this. Telling her that laparoscopy carries a similar wound infection rate as open is factually wrong and also resulted in you losing points.

COMMUNICATION PERSPECTIVES

Elaine's perspective

• Elaine is suspicious.
• She wants an explanation as to why she has not made a full recovery.

SIMPSON AND ELAINE

Elaine is a little suspicious that she may have suffered an avoidable complication of her surgery. Unfortunately, this is a position in which we find many patients in recent years. Honest communication has been identified as the key factor to avoiding conflict and litigation. Also spending time with your patient, taking a personal interest and explaining to patients what to expect, all play key roles in building a rapport with your patient.[8,9]

Halsted's perspective

• If you suggested it was Halsted's fault, he is naturally furious at your suggestion that his surgical ineptitude has resulted in Elaine's wound infection.
• You were not present at the original surgery and could not have appreciated the reasons for the clinical decisions made.
• He is also angry that your lack of surgical knowledge has resulted in a legal letter to the department.

SIMPSON AND HALSTED

Halsted is understandably furious if you told the patient that his lack of skill resulted in a surgical infection, or if you did not know the infection rate in laparoscopic versus open appendectomies. These examples of failed communication have brought embarrassment and legal proceedings against the department. If you do not know the answer to a patient's question, you have an obligation to be honest and explain that you will find the answer for them. This lack of honesty will cost you your relationship with the patient.

What happened to Elaine?

Elaine's wound infection settled relatively quickly once the collection of pus had been drained. She required dressings for several weeks as the wound healed by secondary intention. Overall, she was accepting of the complication and happy with her care; she did not seek compensation.

REFERENCE LIST

1. Cuschieri A. *Clinical Surgery*, 2nd edn. Oxford: Blackwells, 2003.

2. Dunn DC. *Dunn's Surgical Diagnosis and Management*, 3rd edn. Oxford: Blackwells, 1999.

3. Sauerland S, Lefering R, Neugebauer EA. Laparoscopic versus open surgery for suspected appendicitis. Cochrane Database Syst Rev 2004;4:CD001546.

4. Guller U, Hervey S, Purves H, et al. Laparoscopic versus open appendectomy: outcomes comparison based on a large administrative database. Ann Surg 2004;239(1):43–52.

5. Heikkinen TJ, Haukipuro K, Hulkko A. Cost-effective appendectomy. Open or laparoscopic? A prospective randomized study. Surg Endosc 1998;12(10):1204–1208.

6. Macarulla E, Vallet J, Abad JM, Hussein H, Fernandez E, Nieto B. Laparoscopic versus open appendectomy: a prospective randomized trial. Surg Laparosc Endosc 1997;7(4):335–339.

7. Ming PC, Yan TY, Tat LH. Risk factors of postoperative infections in adults with complicated appendicitis. Surg Laparosc Endosc Percutan Tech 2009;19(3):244–248.

8. Correia NG. Adverse events: reducing the risk of litigation. Cleve Clin J Med 2002;69(1):15–4.

9. Levinson W, Roter DL, Mullooly JP, Dull VT, Frankel RM. Physician–patient communication. The relationship with malpractice claims among primary care physicians and surgeons. JAMA 1997;277(7):553–559.

Case perspectives: Al Lopez

THERAPEUTIC PERSPECTIVES

Oxygen

- A number of experimental pneumothorax models have demonstrated an increased rate of lung expansion when supplemental oxygen is administered.[1-3]
- This is likely to be related to supplemental oxygen decreasing the partial pressure of alveolar nitrogen, creating an increased nitrogen gradient between the pleural space and alveolar space. This facilitates the absorption of nitrogen from the pleural space to the alveoli.[4]

SIMPSON AND OXYGEN

Al has a chest injury and is breathless and oxygenating at just 91%, perilously close to the slope of the sigmoid-shaped oxygen desaturation curve. Clearly he needs supplemental oxygen for this reason. However, as seen above, there is evidence that this supplemental oxygen will help his pneumothorax also. Trying to take the history first without oxygen resulted in you being deducted points although Eileen saves the situation by intervening. Taking the history while Al has a face mask on makes it difficult for him to talk while exacerbating the obvious hostility between him and his wife. Although nasal prongs will not deliver as much oxygen as a face mask, they will act as a temporising measure while you take a history. Doing this earned you points.

2 The diagnosis of a tension pneumothorax

- Universal findings in a tension pneumothorax are chest pain and respiratory distress. Common findings (50–75%) are tachycardia and ipsilateral decreased air entry. Inconsistent findings are a low SpO_2, tracheal deviation and hypotension.[5]
- Many of these 'consistent' signs can be found with other common respiratory conditions.
- Generally the patient with a tension pneumothorax will be *in extremis*.[6]
- The diagnosis of a tension pneumothorax on chest x-ray has been associated with a fourfold increase in morbidity related to the time delay to diagnosis.[7,8]

SIMPSON AND TENSION PNEUMOTHORAX

Al does not exhibit the classic presentation of a tension pneumothorax and while certainly exceptions do occur, taking the action of inserting a wide-bore cannula into his chest was not warranted and resulted in you being deducted points.

3 Chest drain

- Second only to fractured ribs, a pneumothorax is the most common sign of chest trauma, occurring in up to 50% of chest trauma victims.[9]
- In half of these cases the pneumothorax may be occult, and as a chest drain is mandatory with positive pressure ventilation, in such patients a CT thorax should be performed.[9]
- While most surgeons will place a chest drain in traumatic pneumothoraces, there is evidence that carefully selected patients may be managed conservatively without a chest drain, with only 9% of these patients eventually requiring drainage.[10]
- In the presence of an associated haemothorax, a chest drain is recommended.[11]

SIMPSON AND CHEST DRAIN

Al has pleuritic chest pain, shortness of breath and is hypoxic. While there is certainly evidence that some patients may not require drainage, clearly he needs a chest drain. Failing to do this resulted in a deduction of points.

4 Flying

- Studies are few and are limited.
- Guidelines suggest that it is safe to fly within 2–3 weeks of a pneumothorax.[12]
- One study specifically looking at this question demonstrated no adverse outcomes in those patients flying after 14 days. However, the study was small, with only 12 patients.[12]

SIMPSON AND FLYING

Although the evidence is weak, there would appear to be no absolute contraindication to Al flying in 4 weeks. Knowledge of this gained you points while getting it wrong lost you points. Being sensible enough to admit you don't know did not result in a loss of points.

COMMUNICATION PERSPECTIVES

Al's perspective

- Al has suffered an injury.
- He is not being supported by his wife although she is with him.

SIMPSON AND AL

While the exact details of what has caused the domestic dispute are not clear, they are not important. Your priority is Al who has suffered significant chest trauma. This is a difficult situation, but if you find that Isabella's presence is making it difficult to treat her husband, it would be prudent to temporarily remove her from the process. If necessary, this should be done with tact so as not to make a difficult situation worse. Asking Isabella to leave for a moment as you must exam her husband and the space is limited is a possible way of achieving this.

Isabella's perspective

- Isabella is clearly angry.
- Their marriage has been difficult for over 1 year.
- Isabella has frequently considered separating from her husband.

SIMPSON AND ISABELLA

You do not know the exact details of Isabella and Al's relationship. Although married for 20 years, their relationship is coming to an end. Your priority is clearly to ensure that Al is diagnosed and treated properly. While you cannot influence what is happening on a social level, you should limit the effect of this on your patient while he is under your care.

What happened to Al?

Al required a chest drain and his lung reinflated over the course of 5 days. Unfortunately, he developed a secondary lung infection and his discharge was delayed. On day 8 he developed chest pain and his ECG demonstrated ST elevation and T-wave inversion consistent with a myocardial infarction. In total he spent 27 days in hospital. Three months later he separated from his wife and they now live apart.

REFERENCE IST

1. England GJ, Hill RC, Timberlake GA, et al. Resolution of experimental pneumothorax in rabbits by graded oxygen therapy. J Trauma 1998;45(2):333–334.

Section 3

2. Hill RC, DeCarlo DP Jr, Hill JF, Beamer KC, Hill ML, Timberlake GA. Resolution of experimental pneumothorax in rabbits by oxygen therapy. Ann Thorac Surg 1995;59(4):825–827.

3. Zierold D, Lee SL, Subramanian S, DuBois JJ. Supplemental oxygen improves resolution of injury-induced pneumothorax. J Pediatr Surg 2000;35(6):998–1001.

4. Courmier Y. The reabsorption of gases from the pleural space. In: Shields TW (ed) General Thoracic Surgery, 4th edn. Philadelphia: Williams &Wilkins, 1994: 657–661.

5. Leigh-Smith S, Harris T. Tension pneumothorax – time for a re-think? Emerg Med J 2005;22(1):8–16.

6. American College of Surgeons. Advanced Trauma Life Support, 8th edn. Chicago: American College of Surgeons, 2009.

7. Steier M, Ching N, Roberts EB, Nealon TF Jr. Pneumothorax complicating continuous ventilatory support. J Thorac Cardiovasc Surg 1974;67(1):17–23.

8. Kollef MH. Risk factors for the misdiagnosis of pneumothorax in the intensive care unit. Crit Care Med 1991;19(7):906–910.

9. Bridges KG, Welch G, Silver M, Schinco MA, Esposito B. CT detection of occult pneumothorax in multiple trauma patients. J Emerg Med 1993;11(2):179–186.

10. Johnson G. Traumatic pneumothorax: is a chest drain always necessary? J Accid Emerg Med 1996;13(3):173–174.

11. Noppen M, de Keukeleire T. Pneumothorax. Respiration 2008;76(2):121–127.

12. Cheatham ML, Safcsak K. Air travel following traumatic pneumothorax: when is it safe? Am Surg 1999;65(12):1160–1164.

INVESTIGATIONS

Name: Lizzie Thurston   MRN: 289876   DOB: 04/08/1984
Adress: Apt. 198 Angels Walk   Loc: Emergency Dept. Pilgrims
Delphi   Sex: F   Phone: Req by: Simpson
Specimen No: PH763967   (Biochemistry)   <PgDn> for later samples

PH763578   13/03/2011   03:27   Whole Blood

WBC	16.9	x10^9/L	(4 to 11)	Auth
RBC	4.55	x10^12/l	(4.5 to 5.3)	Auth
HB	12.2	g/dl	(12 to 16)	Auth
HCT	0.39	l/l	(0.36 to 0.5)	Auth
MCV	93.4	fl	(76 to 96)	Auth
MCH	33.0	pg	(27 to 32)	Auth
MCHC	33.3	g/dl	(32 to 36)	Auth
PLT	290	x10^9/l	(140 to 440)	Auth
Neutrophils	4.80	x10^9/l	(1.8 to 8)	Auth
Lymphocytes	3.10	x10^9/l	(1.5 to 3.5)	Auth
Monocytes	0.54	x10^9/l	(0.16 to 1)	Auth
Eosinophils	0.29	x10^9/l	(0 to 0.5)	Auth
Basophils	0.12	x10^9/l	(0 to 0.2)	Auth

1 Date 2 Earlst 3 Latst 4 rep seQ 5 Spec 6 DFT 7 Matches 8 Options 9 Exit X
No more samples
Disc: HAEM Sect: Haem Pilgrims Emergency department WRNQ/APEX Overtype

---

Name: Lizzie Thurston   MRN: 289876   DOB: 04/08/1984
Adress: Apt. 198 Angels Walk   Loc: Emergency Dept. Pilgrims
Delphi   Sex: F   Phone: Req by: Simpson
Specimen No: PH763678   (Biochemistry)   <PgDn> for later samples

PH763517   13/03/2011   03:27   Whole Blood

Sodium	142	mmol/L	(132 to 144)	Auth
Potassium	3.7	mmol/L	(3.5 to 5.0)	Auth
Chloride	94	mmol/L	(95 to 107)	Auth
Urea	11.0	mmol/L	(2.5 to 7.0)	Auth
Creatinine	98	umol/L	(50 to 130)	Auth
Total Protein	64	g/L	(62 to 82)	Auth
Albumin	35	g/L	(36 to 44)	Auth
AST	16	U/L	(6 to 42)	Auth
ALT	12	U/L	(4 to 45)	Auth
Total Bilirubin	16	umol/L	(2 to 20)	Auth
GGT	27	U/L	(6 to 48)	Auth
Alkaline Phosphatase	98	U/L	(40 to 130)	Auth
Amylase	32	U/L	(28 to 150)	Auth
C-Reactive Protein	76	mg/L	(0 to 10)	Auth
Calcium	2.5	mmol/L	(2.1 to 2.62)	Auth
Haemolysis index	0			

1 Date 2 Earlst 3 Latst 4 rep seQ 5 Spec 6 DFT 7 Matches 8 Options 9 Exit X
Disc: Biochem Sect: Biochem Pilgrims Emergency department WRNQ/APEX
Overtype

Name: Elaine Cardosa
Adress: 2 Arad Drathar Alreha

MRN: 247867   DOB: 09/10/1989
Loc: Emergency Dept. Pilgrims
Sex: F   Phone: Req by: Simpson

Specimen No: PH763623   (Biochemistry)   <PgDn> for later samples

PH763578	13/03/2011	04:10	Whole Blood		
WBC	12.7	×10^9/L	(4 to 11	) Auth
RBC	3.55	×10^12/l	(4.5 to 5.3	) Auth
HB	13.2	g/dl	(12 to 16	) Auth
HCT	0.36	l/l	(0.36 to 0.5	) Auth
MCV	91.5	fl	(76 to 96	) Auth
MCH	28.0	pg	(27 to 32	) Auth
MCHC	34.3	g/dl	(32 to 36	) Auth
PLT	210	×10^9/l	(140 to 440	) Auth
Neutrophils	3.80	×10^9/l	(1.8 to 8	) Auth
Lymphocytes	1.90	×10^9/l	(1.5 to 3.5	) Auth
Monocytes	0.34	×10^9/l	(0.16 to 1	) Auth
Eosinophils	0.33	×10^9/l	(0 to 0.5	) Auth
Basophils	0.09	×10^9/l	(0 to 0.2	) Auth

1 Date 2 Earlst 3 Latst 4 rep seQ 5 Spec 6 DFT 7 Matches 8 Options 9 Exit X
No more samples
Disc: HAEM Sect: Haem Pilgrims Emergency department WRNQ/APEX Overtype

---

Name: Alberto Lopez
Adress: 1089 Raven Walk
     Ursa's place

MRN: 197654   DOB: 23/12/1968
Loc: Emergency Dept, Pilgrims
Sex: M   Phone: Req by: Simpson

Specimen No: PH763987   (Biochemistry)   <PgDn> for later samples

PH763517	13/03/2011	06:37	Arterial Blood	
pH	7.45		(7.36 to 7.44) Auth
pCO2	3.8	kPa	(4.5 to 6.1) Auth
PO2	10	kPa	(11.3 to 14) Auth
Actual Bicarbonate	25	mmol/L	(22 to 26) Auth
Base Excess	1.4	mmol/L	(−2.5 to 2.5) Auth
Oxygen Saturation	93	%	

1 Date 2 Earlst 3 Latst 4 rep seQ 5 Spec 6 DFT 7 Matches 8 Options 9 Exit X
Disc: Biochem Sect: Biochem Pilgrims Emergency department WRNQ/APEX
Overtype

Make A Decision Online

The official website of the 'Make a Decision' series is www.pilgrimshospital.com, here you will find further sample cases including those from other editions. As this book is made up of those cases which have taught us something important in our careers, we encourage you to submit outlines of the cases that have impacted on you, along with the characters that you have encountered (good and bad) along the way. We will try to use both these stories and characters in future editions and if so will acknowledge your contribution. Please follow the instructions on the website to upload your contributions and images. The website also has several other features which you may find helpful including discussions on the main characters and the cases already used, along with further useful links and tips.

A further website which we established some time ago is www.surgent.ie. Possibly one of the most frustrating parts of clinical assessment is that there are no past papers outlining exactly what other students have been assessed on. Surgent was set up to try and remedy this. It is a collection of photographs and cases that we have previously used to assess our own students in their final examinations.

Follow Simpson on twitter as we discuss some difficult cases as they unfold http://twitter.com/drasimpson

Find Dr. Simpson on Facebook. Look for "Dra Simpson"

Podcasts we have found useful

One of the great technological advances of this decade has been the podcast. It is now possible to listen for free, to experts and authors discuss some of the landmark medical issues of our day. While this is not an extensive list by any means, below are some of the podcasts that we have found invaluable to our practice. Further lists are available online through Apples iTunes, and those below can also be accessed in this manner.

1. Cochrane collaboration group at www.cochrane.org

2. MedlinePlus presents a weekly update by the director of the National Library of Medicine, highlighting health news and accompanying information. It is available at www.nlm.nih.gov/medlineplus/directorscomments.html

3. Dr. Jeffrey Guy, director of the burns unit at Vanderbilt University, produces wonderful regular podcasts on a variety of topics, but specialising in critical care. They provide a well researched and easy to follow overview of important topics and can be found at www.burndoc.net/links.html

4. Each week the New England Journal of Medicine releases a podcast highlighting some of their lead articles. Although a little short, it does provide a nice overview of s2ome of their key papers. It can be found at http://content.nejm.org/misc/podcast.dtl

5. A newly established website www.surginfection.com aims to address an incredibly important problem, that of surgical infections. It's author, Dr. Seamus McHugh, delivers regular podcasts discussing some of the relevant literature.